ECG
Interpretation

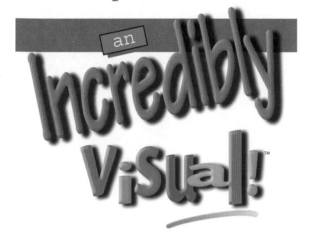

Pocket Guide

ECG
Interpretation

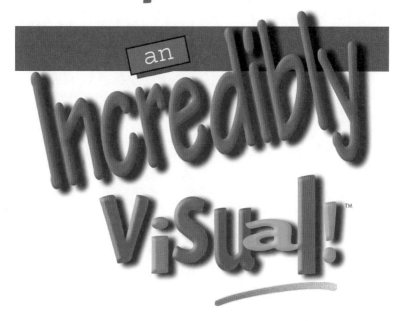

Pocket Guide

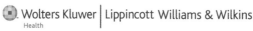

Wolters Kluwer | Lippincott Williams & Wilkins
Health

Philadelphia · Baltimore · New York · London
Buenos Aires · Hong Kong · Sydney · Tokyo

Staff

Executive Publisher
Judith A. Schilling McCann, RN, MSN

Clinical Director
Joan M. Robinson, RN, MSN

Art Director
Elaine Kasmer

Clinical Project Manager
Beverly Ann Tscheschlog, RN, MS

Editors
Diane Labus, Gale Thompson

Copy Editor
Heather Ditch

Illustrator
Bot Roda

Design Assistant
Kate Zulak

Associate Manufacturing Manager
Beth J. Welsh

Editorial Assistants
Karen J. Kirk, Jeri O'Shea, Linda K. Ruhf

Printed in China.

ECGIVPG—010609

ISBN13: 978-1-60547-235-5

Contributors and consultants vi

1 ECG basics 1

2 Rhythm strip interpretation 63

3 Arrhythmias 103

4 Disorder-related ECG changes 191

5 Drug- and electrolyte-related ECG changes 221

6 Pacemakers and the ECG 247

Selected references 277

Index 278

Shelba Durston, RN, MSN, CCRN
Nursing Instructor
San Joaquin Delta College
Stockton, Calif.
Staff Nurse
San Joaquin General Hospital
French Camp, Calif.

Merita Konstantacos, RN, MSN
Nursing Consultant
Clinton, Ohio

Nicolette C. Mininni, RN, MED, CCRN
Advanced Practice Nurse, Critical Care
UPMC Shadyside
Pittsburgh

Pamela Moody, PhD, MSN, APRN-BC, NHA
Nurse Practitioner Consultant
Alabama Department of Public Health
Tuscaloosa

Susan L. Patterson, RN, MS, CCM, ACLS
Faculty, School of Nursing
PRN Staff – Cardiology
Carolinas College Health Sciences, CHS
Charlotte, N.C.

Bruce Austin Scott, MSN, APRN, BC
Nursing Instructor
San Joaquin Delta College
Staff Nurse
St. Joseph's Medical Center
Stockton, Calif.

Allison J. Terry, RN, MSN, PhD
Director of Center for Nursing Workforce Research
Alabama Board of Nursing
Montgomery

Patricia Van Tine, RN, MA
Nursing Faculty
Mt. San Jacinto College
Menifee, Calif.

Wynona Wiggins, RN, MSN, CCRN
Assistant Professor of Nursing
Arkansas State University
State University

Lisa Wolf, RN, MSN
Clinical Educator
Mount Carmel West Hospital
Columbus, Ohio

1

ECG basics

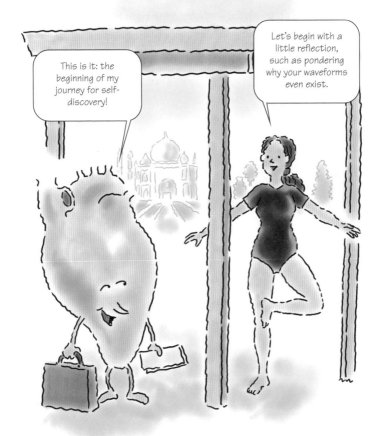

Conduction system

● The heart requires an electrical stimulus to initiate muscle contraction.
● Cardiac cells at rest are considered *polarized* (meaning no electrical activity is taking place).
● After a stimulus occurs, ions cross the cell membrane, causing cell depolarization and myocardial contraction.
● Repolarization occurs as the cell returns to its resting state.
● When depolarization and repolarization occur, the resulting electrical impulse travels through a pathway called the conduction system.

Sinoatrial node

● Located on the endocardial surface of the right atrium
● Acts as the heart's primary pacemaker
● Initiates impulse transmission
● Generates impulses 60 to 100 times per minute (in adults)

(Text continues on page 4.)

A look at atrioventricular node conduction

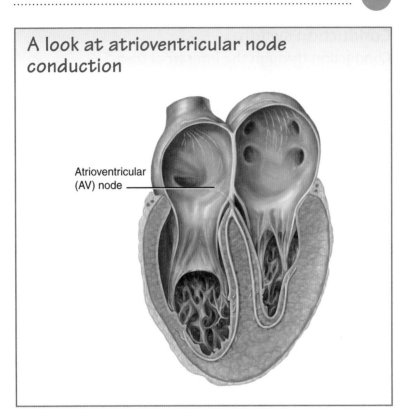

Atrioventricular (AV) node

Conduction system *(continued)*
Conduction through the interatrial tract

- From the SA node, the impulse travels through the left and right atria by way of internodal tracts as well as interatrial tracts (called Bach-mann's bundle).
- This results in atrial contraction.
- The atrial impulse ends at the atrioventricular (AV) node.

> Impulse transmission through the right and left atria occurs so rapidly that the atria contract almost simultaneously.

(Text continues on page 6.)

The atrial conduction system

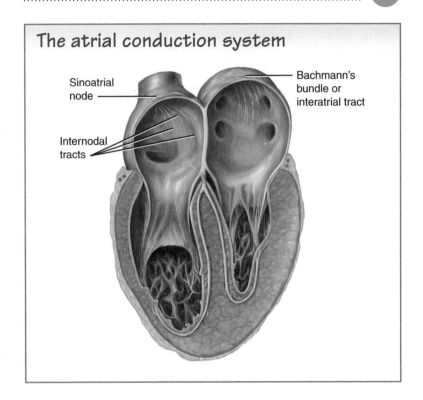

Sinoatrial node

Bachmann's bundle or interatrial tract

Internodal tracts

Conduction system *(continued)*

AV node

- Located in the atrial septal wall
- Delays impulses to allow time for the ventricles to completely fill with blood before they contract
- Has its own pacemaker ability with a firing rate of 40 to 60 times per minute
- Only initiates an impulse if it does not receive one from higher in the atria

Ventricular conduction

- Impulses travel from the AV node through the ventricles by way of the bundle of His, the left and right bundle branches, and, finally, the Purkinje fibers.
- Purkinje fibers extend deep in the myocardial tissue.
  - These fibers can also serve as a pacemaker.
  - They can discharge impulses at a rate of 20 to 40 times per minute.
  - They only fire when they fail to receive an impulse from a higher pacemaker.

The ventricular conduction system

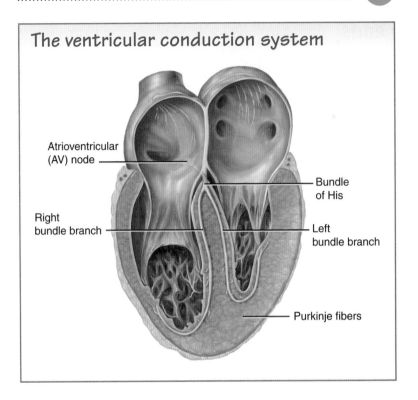

Atrioventricular (AV) node

Bundle of His

Right bundle branch

Left bundle branch

Purkinje fibers

Leads

● Leads provide a view of the heart's electrical activity between one positive pole and one negative pole.
● Between the two poles lies an imaginary line representing the lead's *axis* (the direction in which the current is moving through the heart).
● Each lead generates its own characteristic tracing.
● The direction of the electric current determines how the waveform appears on the ECG tracing.
  – Current moving toward the positive pole produces a waveform that's deflected upward (positive deflection).
  – Current moving away from the positive pole produces a waveform that's deflected downward (negative deflection).
  – Current flowing perpendicular to the axis produces a waveform that may be unusually small or that goes both directions.
  – When electrical activity is absent or too small to measure, the waveform is a straight line (also called an *isoelectric deflection*).

(Text continues on page 10.)

Identifying waveform deflection

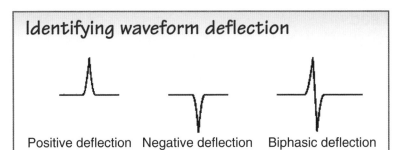

Positive deflection   Negative deflection   Biphasic deflection

Leads (continued)
Bipolar leads

- Require a positive and a negative electrode for monitoring
- Use a third electrode, which acts as the ground
- Include limb leads I, II, and III

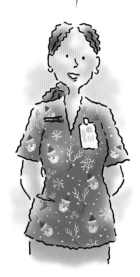

The ground electrode helps prevent electrical interference from appearing on the ECG recording.

(Text continues on page 12.)

A look at the bipolar leads

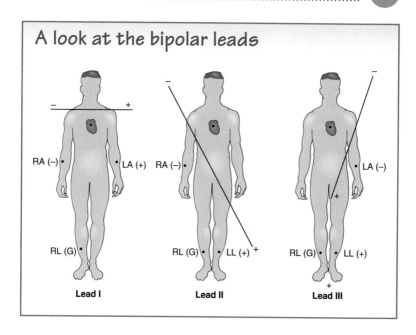

Lead I

Lead II

Lead III

Leads (continued)

Unipolar leads

● Use only a positive electrode
● Use the heart's center as the negative pole, which is calculated by the ECG machine
● Include the augmented leads aV_R, aV_L, and aV_F and the precordial leads

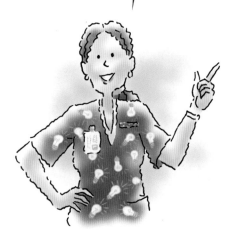

A look at the unipolar leads

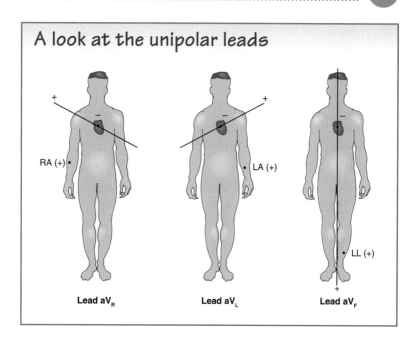

Lead aV_R   Lead aV_L   Lead aV_F

Planes

- A plane is a cross-section of the heart.
- They offer an alternative view of the heart's electrical activity.

Frontal plane

- Formed by dividing the heart vertically from top to bottom
- Views electrical activity from anterior to posterior
- Provides a view of the six limb leads

Horizontal plane

- Formed by dividing the heart into upper and lower portions
- Views electrical activity from a superior or an inferior approach
- Provides a view of the six precordial leads

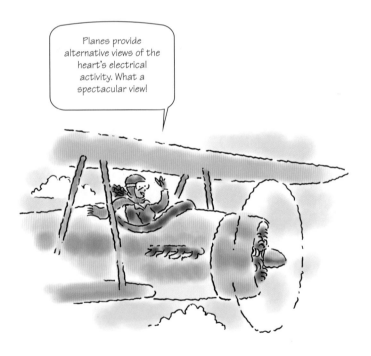

A view of the heart's planes

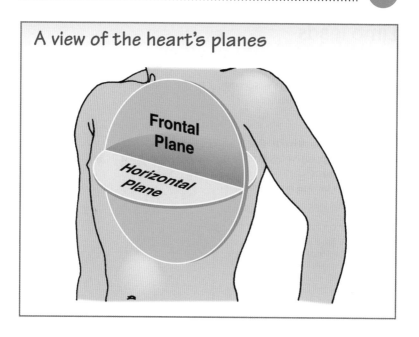

Limb leads

● Each limb lead transmits information about a different area of the left ventricle.
● Waveform shape varies according to the relationship of the lead to the wave of depolarization.

Lead I

● Produces a positive deflection
● Requires a positive electrode on the left arm and a negative electrode on the right arm
● Views the lateral heart wall

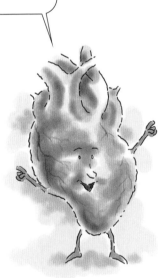

Think of an ECG like positive thinking. Just as positive thoughts may attract good things, current flows away from the negative and toward the positive!

(Text continues on page 18.)

A look at lead I

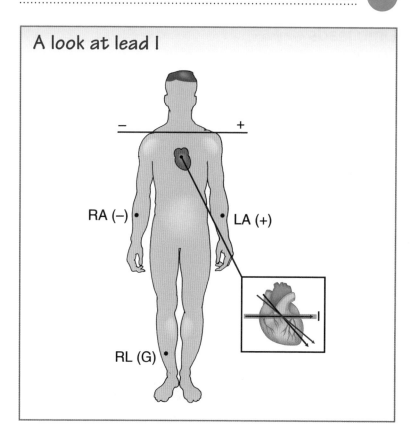

Limb leads *(continued)*
Lead II

- Produces a positive deflection
- Requires a positive electrode on the left leg and a negative electrode on the right arm
- Views the inferior heart wall

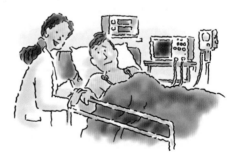

Lead II is commonly used for routine monitoring. It's also useful for detecting sinus node and atrial arrhythmias and monitoring the inferior wall of the left ventricle.

(Text continues on page 20.)

A look at lead II

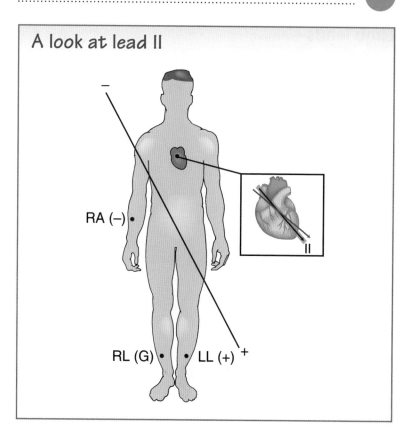

RA (−) •

RL (G) •   • LL (+) +

Limb leads *(continued)*
Lead III

- Produces a positive deflection
- Requires a positive electrode on the left leg and a negative electrode on the left arm
- Views the inferior heart wall

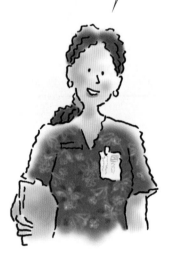

Just like lead II, lead III also helps detect changes associated with the inferior wall of the left ventricle.

(Text continues on page 22.)

A look at lead III

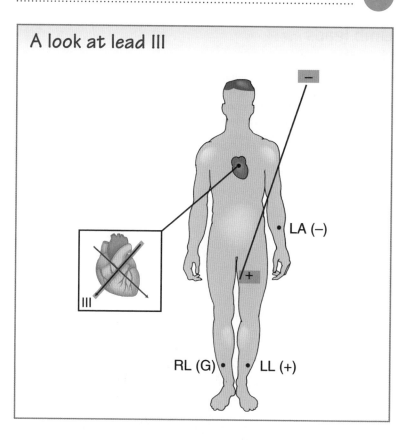

Limb leads *(continued)*

Lead aV_R
- Stands for "augments voltage right"
- Measures impulses flowing from the heart to the right arm
- Produces a negative deflection
- Requires a positive electrode on the right arm
- Provides no interpretive data

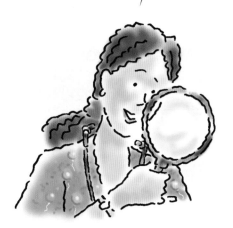

These leads are called "augmented" because the small waveforms that normally would appear from these unipolar leads are enhanced by the ECG.

(Text continues on page 24.)

A look at lead aV$_R$

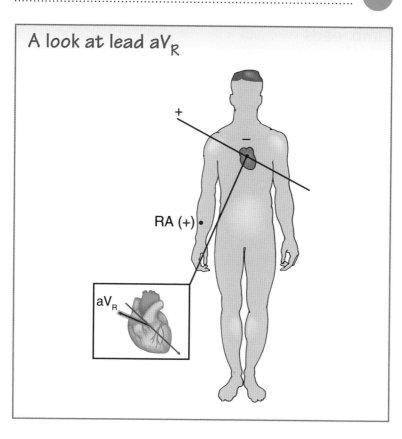

+

−

RA (+) •

aV$_R$

Limb leads *(continued)*

Lead aV$_L$

- Stands for "augmented voltage left"
- Measures impulses flowing from the heart to the left arm
- Produces a positive deflection
- Requires a positive electrode on the left arm
- Provides a view of the lateral heart wall

(Text continues on page 26.)

A look at lead aV_L

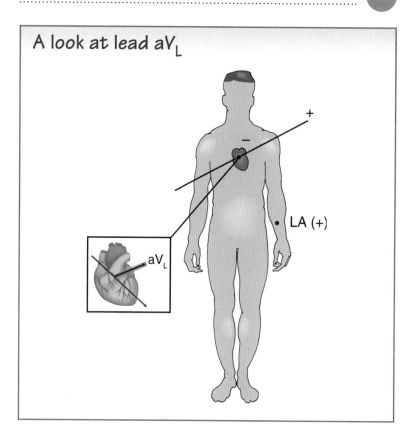

Limb leads *(continued)*
Lead aV_F

- Stands for "augmented voltage foot"
- Measures impulses flowing from the heart to the left leg
- Produces a positive deflection
- Requires a positive electrode on the left leg
- Provides a view of the inferior heart wall

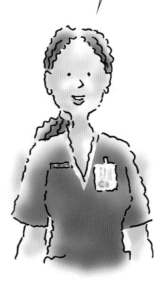

The three augmented limb leads also provide a view of the heart's frontal plane.

A look at lead aV_F

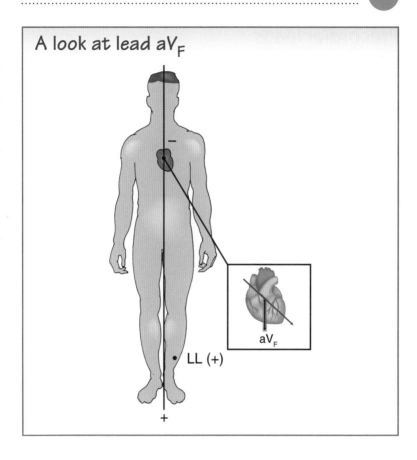

Precordial leads

- Includes six chest leads
- Uses only unipolar leads
- Requires precise lead positioning for an accurate tracing

Lead V_1

- Produces a negative deflection
- Requires placement of a positive electrode on the right side of the sternum at fourth intercostal rib space
- Provides a view of the anteroseptal heart wall

(Text continues on page 30.)

Examining lead V₁

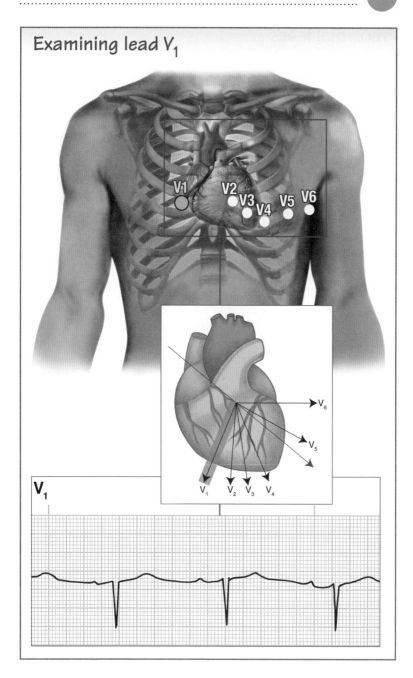

Precordial leads *(continued)*

Lead V$_2$

- Produces a negative deflection
- Requires placement of an electrode to the left of the sternum at the fourth intercostal space
- Provides a view of the anteroseptal heart wall

(Text continues on page 32.)

Examining lead V₂

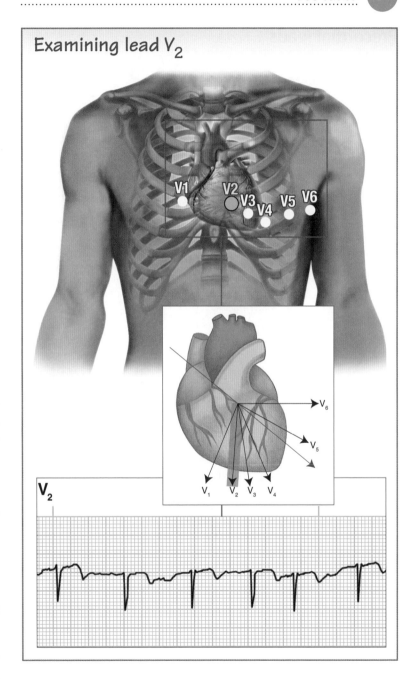

Precordial leads (continued)

Lead V$_3$

- Produces a biphasic deflection
- Requires placement of an electrode between V$_2$ and V$_4$ at the fifth intercostal space
- Provides views of the anterior and anteroseptal heart walls

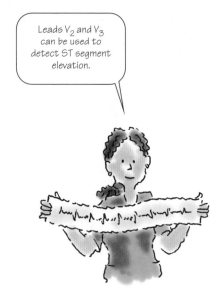

(Text continues on page 34.)

Examining lead V₃

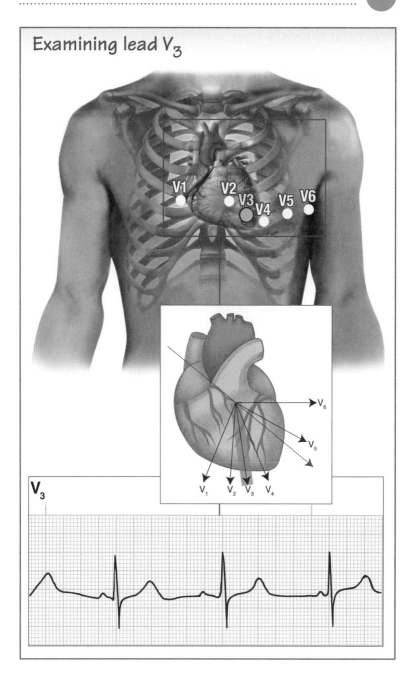

Precordial leads *(continued)*

Lead V$_4$

- Produces a positive deflection
- Requires placement of an electrode at the fifth intercostal space at the midclavicular line
- Provides a view of the anterior heart wall

(Text continues on page 36.)

Examining lead V₄

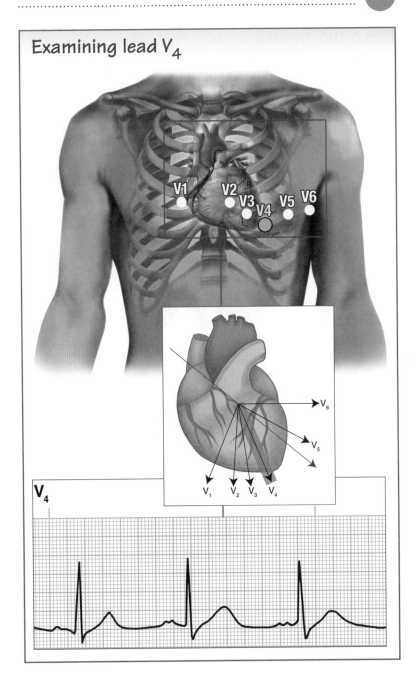

Precordial leads *(continued)*
Lead V₅

- Produces a positive deflection
- Requires placement of an electrode at the fifth intercostal space anterior to the axillary line
- Provides a view of the lateral heart wall

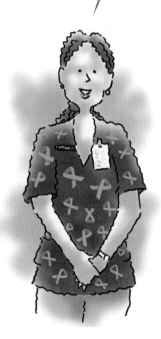

Along with lead V₄, lead V₅ can show changes in the ST-segment or T-wave.

(Text continues on page 38.)

Examining lead V₅

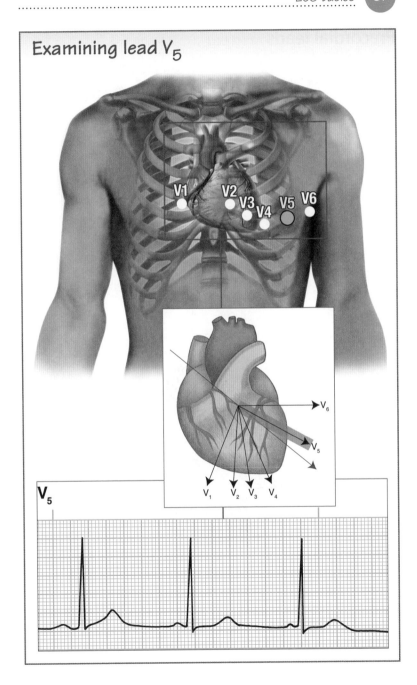

V₅

Precordial leads *(continued)*
Lead V₆

- Produces a positive deflection
- Requires placement of an electrode at the fifth intercostal space at the midaxillary line
- Provides a view of the lateral heart wall

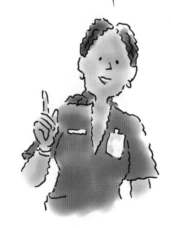

That's right; the electrode for lead V₆ is placed in the fifth intercostal space, just like the electrodes for leads V₄ and V₅.

Examining lead V₆

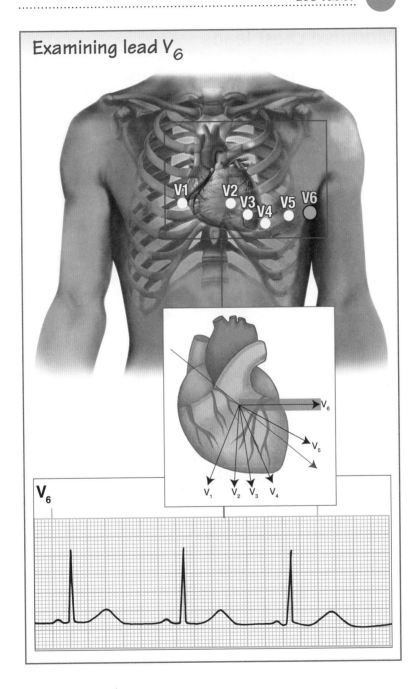

Modified chest leads

- Represented by the initials "MCL"
- Requires placement of a negative electrode on the left side of the chest (rather than having the center of the heart function as the negative lead)

MCL$_1$

- Can be used to assess QRS complex arrhythmias, premature ventricular beats, and to distinguish types of tachycardia
- Can also be used to assess bundle-branch defects and P-wave changes and to confirm pacemaker wire placement

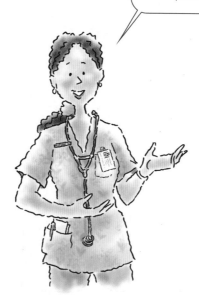

When the positive electrode is on the right side of the heart and the electrical current travels toward the left ventricle, the waveform has a negative deflection. As a result, ectopic or abnormal beats deflect in a positive direction.

(Text continues on page 42.)

A look at MCL₁

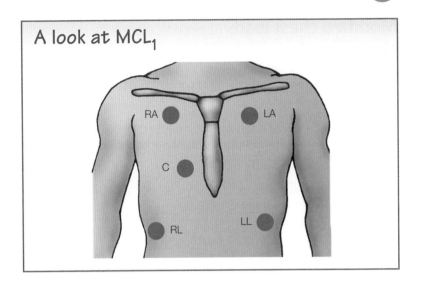

Modified chest leads (continued)
MCL$_6$

- May be used as an alternative to MCL$_1$
- Most closely approximates the ECG pattern produced by the chest lead V$_6$
- Monitors ventricular conduction changes
- Requires placement of a positive electrode at the midaxillary line of the fifth intercostal space, a negative electrode below the left shoulder, and a ground below the right shoulder

MCL$_6$ provides a pretty good picture of ventricular conduction changes.

A look at MCL₆

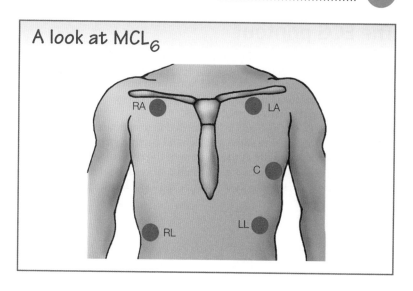

The ECG printout

● Waveforms produced by the heart's electrical current are recorded on graph paper by a heated stylus.

● ECG paper consists of vertical and horizontal lines that form a grid.

● The grid allows measurement of the size and frequency of wave complexes for comparison to normal ranges.

● On a 12-lead ECG, the leads are recorded in a standard order.

● The ECG recording will show a 10 second rhythm strip (obtained from lead II or V_1), usually at the bottom of the recording.

● The ECG recording also contains lead markers, lead names, and standardization marks, which are normally 10 small squares in height.

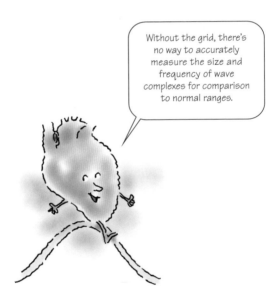

Without the grid, there's no way to accurately measure the size and frequency of wave complexes for comparison to normal ranges.

(Text continues on page 46.)

A look at an ECG printout

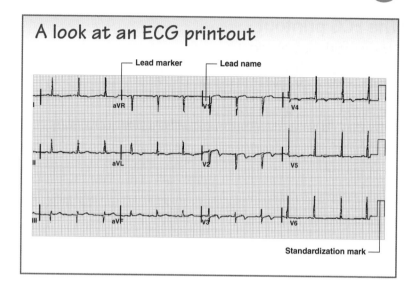

Lead marker

Lead name

Standardization mark

The ECG printout *(continued)*
Horizontal axis blocks

- The horizontal axis of the ECG represents time.
- Each small block equals 0.04 second.
- Five small blocks form a large block, which equals 0.20 second.
- Five large blocks equal 1 second.
- The time elapsed is calculated based on the number of blocks between two points.

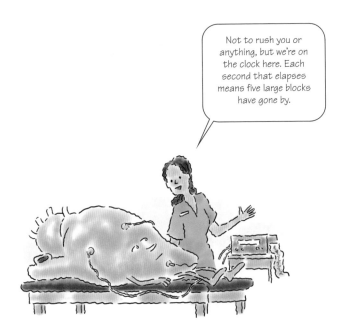

Not to rush you or anything, but we're on the clock here. Each second that elapses means five large blocks have gone by.

(Text continues on page 48.)

Understanding horizontal axis blocks

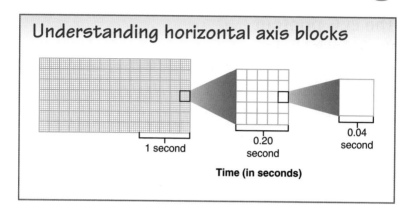

1 second

0.20 second

0.04 second

Time (in seconds)

The ECG printout (continued)

Vertical axis blocks

- The ECG strip's vertical axis measures amplitude in millimeters or electrical voltage in millivolts.
- Each small block represents 1 millimeter or 0.1 millivolt.
- Each large block represents 5 millimeters or 0.5 millivolts.
- The amplitude of a wave, segment, or interval is determined by counting the number of small blocks from the baseline to the highest or lowest point of the wave, segment, or interval.

Understanding vertical axis blocks

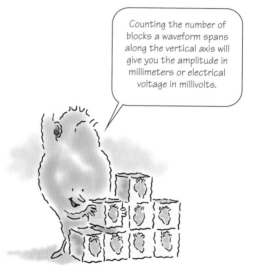

Counting the number of blocks a waveform spans along the vertical axis will give you the amplitude in millimeters or electrical voltage in millivolts.

Identifying monitor problems

- Abnormal waveforms could indicate problems with the monitor.
- Always assess the patient before troubleshooting the equipment.

Artifact

- Also called *waveform interference*
- May result from excessive movement, such as when the patient is experiencing chills, seizures, or anxiety
- Other causes:
  - Dirty or corroded connections
  - Improper application of lead wires or electrodes
  - A short circuit in the cable
  - Electrical interference from other equipment in the room
  - Static electricity from inadequate room humidity

(Text continues on page 52.)

Identifying artifact

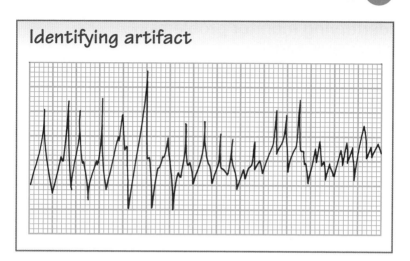

Waveform interference, or artifact, can result from a number of different causes, including excessive patient movement due to chills, seizures, or anxiety.

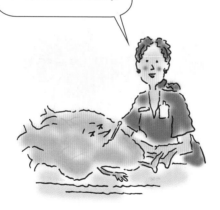

Identifying monitor problems *(continued)*
False high-rate alarm
- May result if the gain setting is set too high (especially in lead MCL_1)
- May also result if the HIGH alarm setting is set too low or the LOW alarm setting is set too high

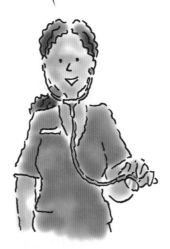

Even if an alarm sounds repeatedly, never just assume it's the equipment. Always assess the patient first.

(Text continues on page 54.)

Identifying a false high-rate alarm

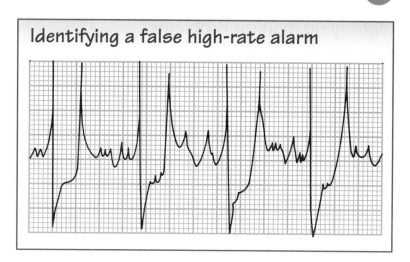

Identifying monitor problems (continued)
Weak signals

- May result from improper electrode application
- Occur if the QRS complex is too small to register
- Can result from wire or cable failure

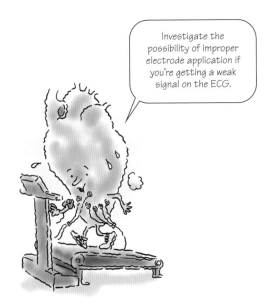

Investigate the possibility of improper electrode application if you're getting a weak signal on the ECG.

(Text continues on page 56.)

Identifying a weak signal

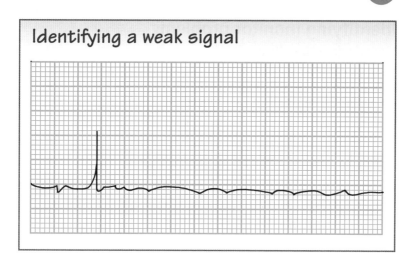

Identifying monitor problems *(continued)*
Wandering baseline

- May occur when the patient is restless
- May reflect chest wall movement during respiration
- Can result if electrodes are positioned over bone

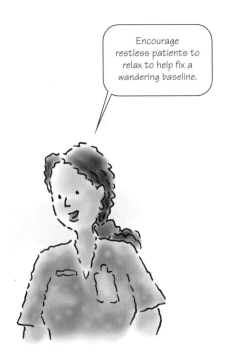

Encourage restless patients to relax to help fix a wandering baseline.

(Text continues on page 58.)

Identifying a wandering baseline

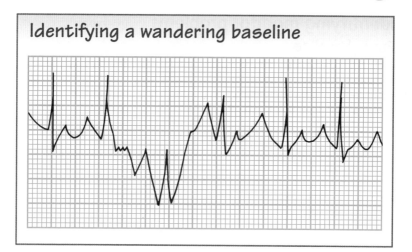

Identifying monitor problems *(continued)*
Fuzzy baseline

- Can occur because of electrical interference from other equipment in the room
- May appear if the patient's bed is improperly grounded
- May signal a malfunctioning electrode

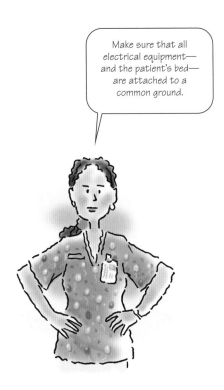

Make sure that all electrical equipment—and the patient's bed—are attached to a common ground.

(Text continues on page 60.)

Identifying a fuzzy baseline

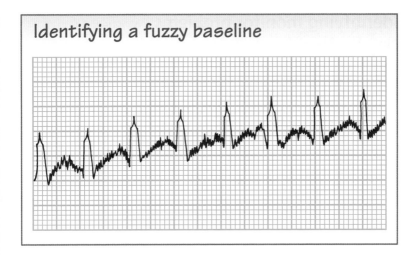

Identifying monitor problems (continued)
No waveform

- Can result from a disconnected electrode
- May occur because of a dry electrode gel
- May signal wire or cable failure
- May occur because of improper electrode placement (perpendicular to the axis of the heart)

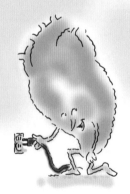

No waveform?
No problem . . .
Before you panic,
check disconnected wires,
cables, or electrodes first.

Identifying no waveform

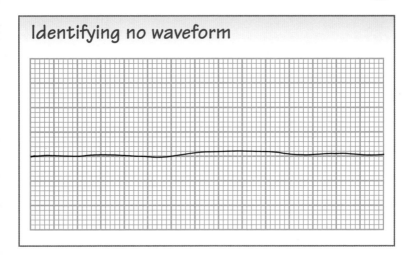

2

Rhythm strip interpretation

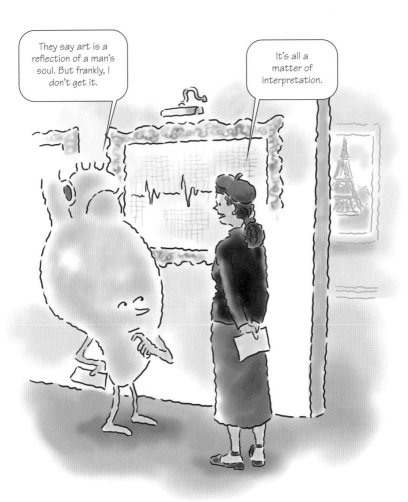

ECG complex

- An electrocardiogram (ECG) complex represents the electrical events occurring in one cardiac cycle.
- A complex consists of five waveforms labeled with the letters P, Q, R, S, and T.
- The middle three letters—Q, R, and S—are referred to as a unit, the QRS complex.
- ECG tracings represent the conduction of electrical impulses from the atria to the ventricles.

(Text continues on page 66.)

ECG waveform components

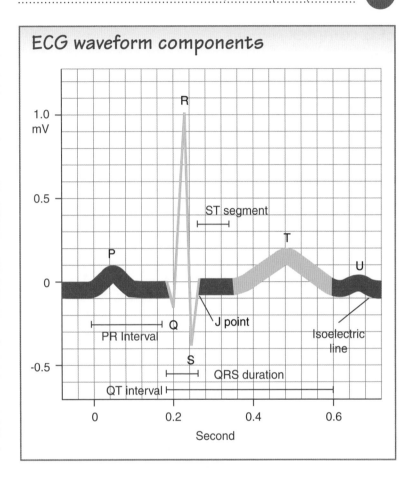

ECG complex *(continued)*
P wave

- Represents atrial depolarization—conduction of an electrical impulse through the atria
- Precedes the QRS complex
- Has an amplitude of 2 to 3 mm high
- Lasts 0.06 to 0.12 second
- Is usually rounded and upright
- Must be upright in leads II and aVF and inverted in lead aVR to be called sinus rhythm

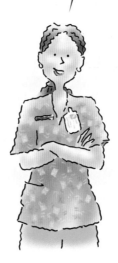

Keep in mind that the ECG records electrical activity only, not mechanical activity or contraction.

(Text continues on page 68.)

Identifying a P wave

ECG complex *(continued)*
PR interval

- Tracks the atrial impulse from the atria through the AV node, bundle of His, and the right and left bundle branches
- Measured from the start of the P wave to start of the QRS complex
- Lasts 0.12 to 0.20 second

(Text continues on page 70.)

Identifying the PR interval

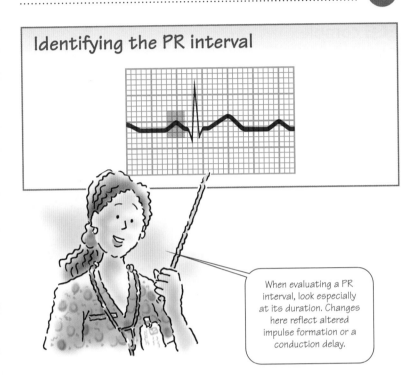

When evaluating a PR interval, look especially at its duration. Changes here reflect altered impulse formation or a conduction delay.

ECG complex *(continued)*
QRS complex

- Represents depolarization of and impulse conduction through the ventricles
- Includes the Q wave (first negative deflection or deflection from the baseline after the P wave), the R wave (the first positive deflection after the Q wave), and the S wave (the first negative deflection after the R wave)
- Measured from the beginning of the Q wave to the end of the S wave (or from the beginning of the R wave if the Q wave is absent)
- Lasts 0.06 to 0.10 second or one-half of the PR interval
- Has an amplitude of 5 to 30 mm high, but differs in each lead

(Text continues on page 72.)

Identifying a QRS complex

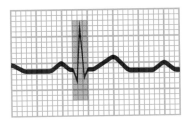

Contrary to popular belief, finding the QRS complex isn't all that complex. Find the p wave, and then follow the wave form down, then up, then down again.

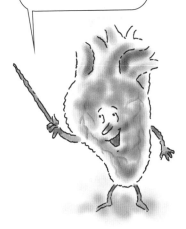

ECG complex *(continued)*
QRS complex *(continued)*
QRS waveform variety

- Various configurations of the QRS complex can occur.
- When documenting a QRS complex, use uppercase letters to indicate a wave with normal or high amplitude (greater than 5 mm).
- Use lower case letters to indicate a QRS complex with a low amplitude (less than 5 mm).

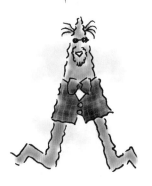

Don't be too quick to judge what's "normal." We QRS complexes like a little variety.

(Text continues on page 74.)

A look at QRS waveforms

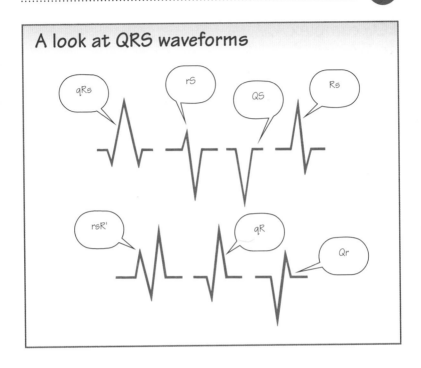

ECG complex (continued)

ST segment

- Represents the end of ventricular depolarization and the start of ventricular recovery or repolarization
- Begins at the J point (which marks the end of the QRS complex)
- Extends to the start of the T wave
- Usually is isoelectric (neither positive or negative in deflection) or on the baseline; may vary from −0.5 to +1 mm in some precordial leads

(Text continues on page 76.)

Identifying an ST segment

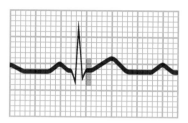

The ST segment begins at the end of the QRS complex and extends to the start of the T wave.

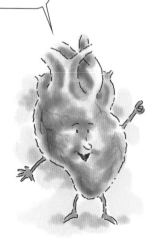

ECG complex *(continued)*

ST segment *(continued)*

ST-segment changes

● An ST segment is considered depressed when it's 0.5 mm or more below the baseline.

● A depressed ST segment may indicate myocardial ischemia or digoxin toxicity.

● An ST segment is considered elevated when it's 1 mm or more above the baseline.

● An elevated ST segment may indicate myocardial injury.

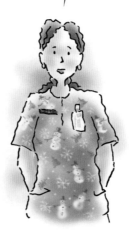

Watch closely for ST-segment changes. Doing so can help you detect myocardial ischemia or injury before infarction develops.

(Text continues on page 78.)

Recognizing ST-segment changes

ST-segment depression

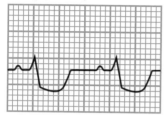

ST-segment elevation

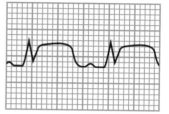

ECG complex *(continued)*

T wave

● Represents the relative refractory period of repolarization or ventricular recovery
● Follows the ST segment
● Has an amplitude of 0.5 mm in leads I, II, and III, and up to 10 mm in the precordial leads
● Typically appears rounded and smooth

> Says here that
> T waves are typically
> rounded and smooth.
> I'm stoked!

(Text continues on page 80.)

Identifying a T wave

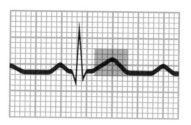

ECG complex *(continued)*
QT interval

- Measures the time needed for ventricular depolarization and repolarization
- Varies with heart rate: a faster heart rate = a shorter QT interval
- Extends from the beginning of the QRS complex to the end of the T wave
- Lasts 0.36 to 0.44 second and can vary with age and gender
- Should not be greater than half the distance between two consecutive R waves

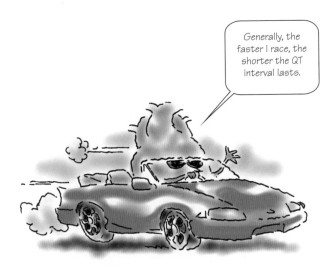

Generally, the faster I race, the shorter the QT interval lasts.

(Text continues on page 82.)

Identifying the QT interval

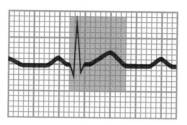

ECG complex *(continued)*

U wave

- Represents repolarization of the His-Purkinje system
- May not appear on an ECG
- Follows the T wave
- Typically appears upright and rounded
- If prominent, may indicate hypercalcemia, hypokalemia, or digoxin toxicity

Identifying a U wave

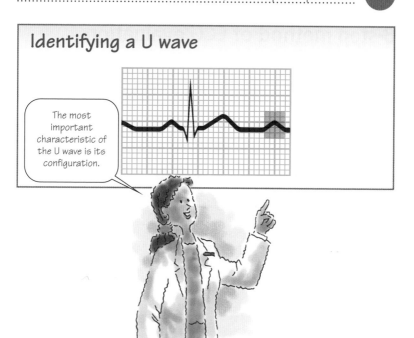

The most important characteristic of the U wave is its configuration.

8-step method of ECG evaluation

- Analyzing a rhythm strip is a skill developed through practice.
- You can use one of several methods, as long as you're consistent.
- Rhythm strip analysis requires a sequential and systematic approach, such as the eight steps outlined here.

Step 1: Determine the rhythm

- For atrial rhythm, measure the P-P interval or the interval between two consecutive P waves.
- Use calipers to measure the interval between the P waves in several ECG cycles.
- The P wave should occur at regular intervals with only small variations associated with respiration.
- For ventricular rhythm, measure the intervals between two consecutive R waves in the QRS complexes.
- If the R-R intervals remain consistent, the ventricular rhythm is regular.

(Text continues on page 86.)

Evaluating atrial and ventricular rhythms

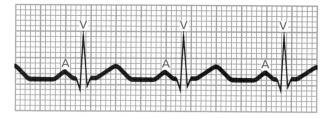

8-step method of ECG evaluation *(continued)*
Step 2: Determine the rate

● If the heart rate is regular, determine the atrial rate by counting the number of small squares between identical points on two consecutive P waves.
● Divide that number by 1,500 to get the atrial rate.
● To determine the ventricular rate, use the same method with two consecutive R waves.

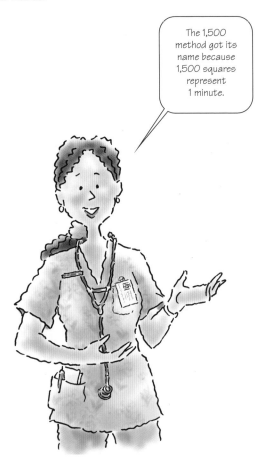

The 1,500 method got its name because 1,500 squares represent 1 minute.

(Text continues on page 88.)

Determining atrial and ventricular rates

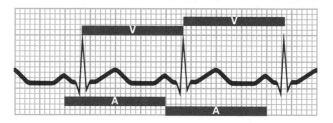

8-step method of ECG evaluation (continued)
Step 3: Evaluate the P wave

● Observe the P wave's size, shape, and location in the waveform.
● If each QRS complex has a P wave, then the sinoatrial (SA) node is initiating the electrical impulse, which it should be.

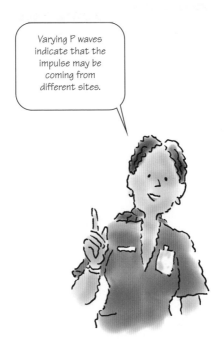

Varying P waves indicate that the impulse may be coming from different sites.

(Text continues on page 90.)

Evaluating the P wave

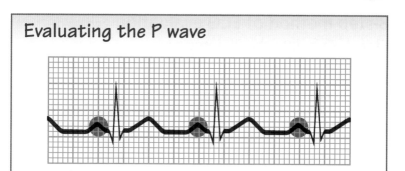

8-step method of ECG evaluation *(continued)*
Step 4: Calculate the PR interval

● Count the number of small squares between the beginning of the
P wave and the beginning of the QRS complex.
● Multiply the number of squares by 0.04 second.
● The normal interval is between 0.12 and 0.2 second, or between 3 and
5 small squares.

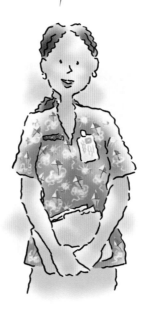

(Text continues on page 92.)

Calculating the PR interval

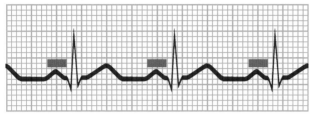

8-step method of ECG evaluation *(continued)*
Step 5: Calculate the duration of the QRS complex

● Count the number of squares between the beginning and the end of the QRS complex.

● Multiply that number by 0.04 second.

● A normal QRS complex is less than 0.12 second or less than 3 small squares wide.

● Check to see if the QRS complexes are the same size and shape.

● Note whether a QRS complex appears after every P wave.

(Text continues on page 94.)

Calculating the duration of the QRS complex

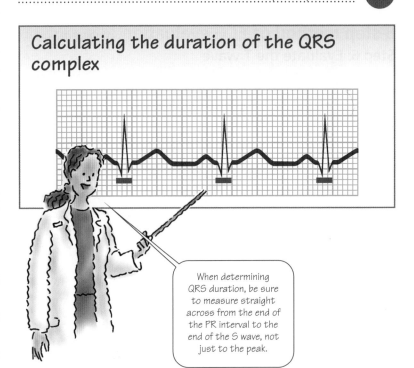

8-step method of ECG evaluation *(continued)*
Step 6: Evaluate the T wave

- Check that the T waves are present and have a normal shape, normal amplitude, and the same deflection as QRS complexes.
- Consider whether a P wave could be hidden in a T wave by looking for extra bumps in the waveform.

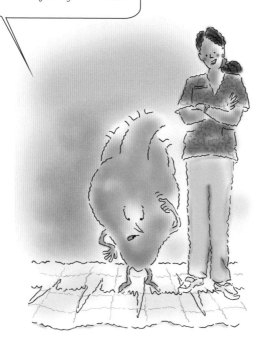

I'm looking for extra bumps that could signify hidden P waves, but all I see are normally configured T waves.

(Text continues on page 96.)

Evaluating the T wave

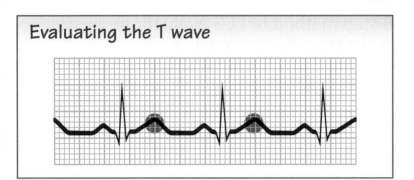

8-step method of ECG evaluation *(continued)*
Step 7: Determine the QT interval

● Count the number of squares from the beginning of the QRS complex to the end of the T wave.
● Multiply this number by 0.04 second.
● The normal range is 0.36 to 0.44 second, or 9 to 11 small squares.

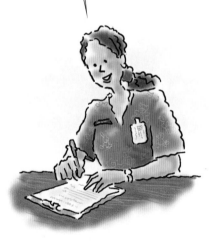

A prolonged QT interval indicates that ventricular repolarization time is slowed. This change may also be associated with certain medications, such as class I antiarrhythmics.

(Text continues on page 98.)

Calculating the duration of the QT interval

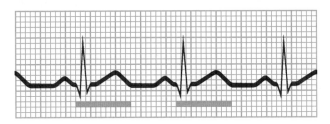

8-step method of ECG evaluation *(continued)*
Step 8: Evaluate other components

● Look for ectopic beats, aberrantly conducted beats, or other abnormalities.

● Make sure the waveform doesn't reflect problems with the monitor.

● Next, check the ST segment for abnormalities and look for a U wave.

● Finally, classify the rhythm strip according to the following characteristics:

    – *Site of rhythm origin:* sinus node, atria, AV node, or ventricles

    – *Rate:* normal (60 to 100 beats/minute), bradycardic (less than 60 beats/minute), or tachycardic (more than 100 beats/minute)

    – *Rhythm:* regular or irregular (which could reflect flutter, fibrillation, heart block, escape, other arrhythmias)

Checking for other abnormalities

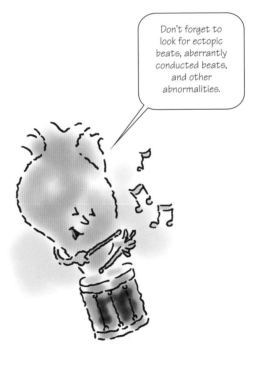

Don't forget to look for ectopic beats, aberrantly conducted beats, and other abnormalities.

Normal sinus rhythm

● Normal sinus rhythm is the standard against which all other rhythms are compared.

● Normal sinus rhythm records an impulse that progresses from the SA node to the ventricles through the normal conduction pathway.

● To be classified as normal sinus rhythm, the:
  – atrial and ventricular rhythm should be regular
  – rate should be between 60 and 100 beats/minute, the SA node's normal firing rate.

Recognizing normal sinus rhythm

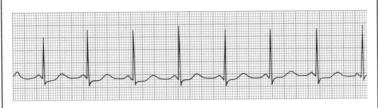

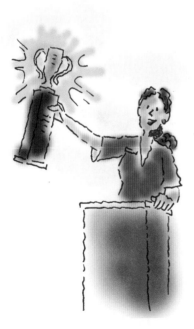

Normal sinus rhythm ... the standard against which all other ECG rhythms are compared!

3 Arrhythmias

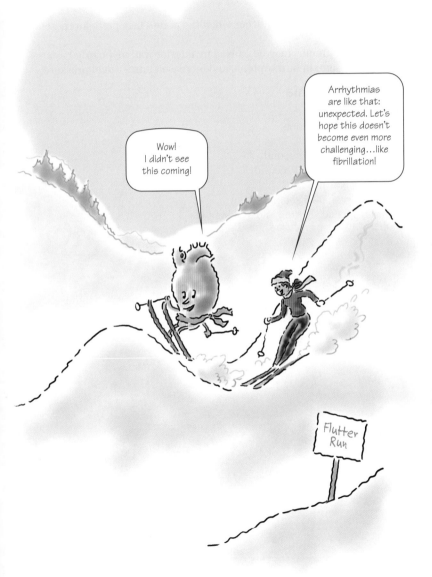

Sinus node arrhythmias

- When the heart functions normally, the SA node, also called the sinus node, acts as the primary pacemaker.
- The SA node assumes this role because its automatic firing rate (60 to 100 beats/minute in an adult at rest) exceeds that of the heart's other pacemakers.
- Sinus node arrhythmias occur when the node's firing rate increases or decreases.
- These arrhythmias may be caused by inferior-wall myocardial infarction, use of digoxin or morphine, and increased intracranial pressure.

Sinus arrhythmia

- *Rhythm*: Irregular
- *Rate*: 70 beats/minute
- *P wave*: Normal
- *PR interval*: 0.16 second
- *QRS complex*: 0.06 second
- *T wave*: Normal
- *QT interval*: 0.36 second
- *Other*: Phasic slowing and quickening

(Text continues on page 106.)

Recognizing sinus arrhythmia

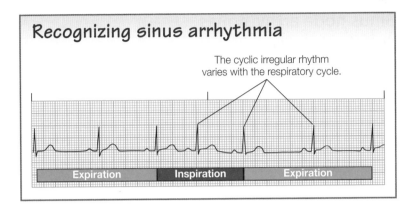

The cyclic irregular rhythm varies with the respiratory cycle.

Expiration | Inspiration | Expiration

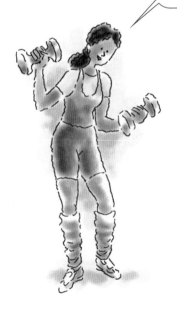

Sinus arrhythmia can occur normally in athletes, children, and older adults, but it rarely occurs in infants.

Sinus node arrhythmias *(continued)*
Sinus bradycardia

- *Rhythm*: Regular
- *Rate*: 50 beats/minute
- *P wave*: Normal
- *PR interval*: 0.16 second
- *QRS complex*: 0.08 second
- *T wave*: Normal
- *QT interval*: 0.50 second

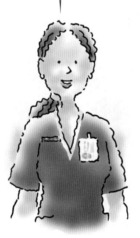

The significance of sinus bradycardia depends upon the symptoms and the underlying cause.

(Text continues on page 108.)

Recognizing sinus bradycardia

A normal P wave precedes each QRS complex.

The rhythm is regular, with a rate below 60 beats/minute.

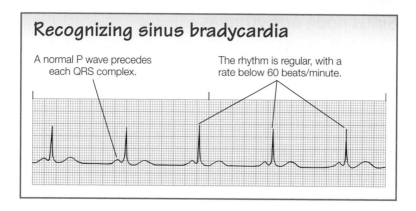

Sinus node arrhythmias *(continued)*
Sinus tachycardia

- *Rhythm*: Regular
- *Rate*: 120 beats/minute
- *P wave*: Normal
- *PR interval*: 0.14 second
- *QRS complex*: 0.06 second
- *T wave*: Normal
- *QT interval*: 0.34 second

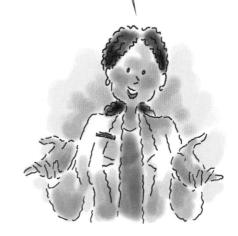

Sinus tachycardia may be a normal response to exercise or high emotional states. On the other hand, persistent tachycardia can lower cardiac output by reducing ventricular filling time and stroke volume.

(Text continues on page 110.)

Recognizing sinus tachycardia

A normal P wave precedes each QRS complex.

The rhythm is regular, with a rate above 100 beats/minute.

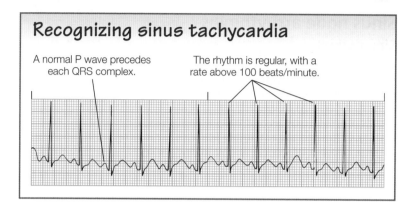

Sinus node arrhythmias *(continued)*
Sinus arrest

- *Rhythm*: Regular, except for the missing PQRST complexes
- *Rate*: Underlying rhythm 100 beats/minute
- *P wave*: Normal; missing during pause
- *PR interval*: 0.20 second
- *QRS complex*: 0.08 second; absent during pause
- *T wave*: Normal; absent during pause
- *QT interval*: 0.40 second; absent during pause

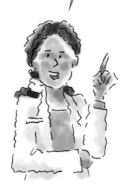

Atrial standstill is called sinus pause when one or two beats aren't formed and sinus arrest when three or more beats aren't formed.

(Text continues on page 112.)

Recognizing sinus arrest

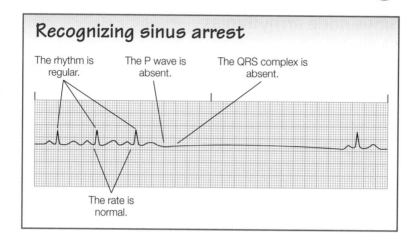

The rhythm is regular.

The P wave is absent.

The QRS complex is absent.

The rate is normal.

Sinus node arrhythmias *(continued)*
SA block

● *Rhythm*: Regular, except during a pause (irregular as a result of the pause)
● *Rate*: Usually within normal limits (60 to 100 beats/minute) before pause
● *P wave*: Periodically absent with entire PQRST complex missing; when present, normal size and configuration and precedes each QRS complex
● *PR interval*: 0.16 second
● *QRS complex*: 0.08 second; absent during pause
● *T wave*: Normal; missing during pause
● *QT interval*: 0.40 second; missing during pause
● *Other*: Entire PQRST complex missing; pause ends with sinus rhythm

(Text continues on page 114.)

Recognizing SA block

Sinoatrial exit block

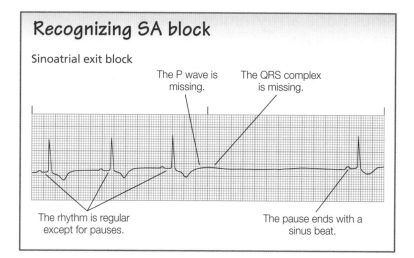

The P wave is missing.

The QRS complex is missing.

The rhythm is regular except for pauses.

The pause ends with a sinus beat.

Sinus node arrhythmias *(continued)*
Sick sinus syndrome

- *Rhythm*: Regular
- *Rate*: Atrial—60 beats/minute; ventricular—70 beats/minute
- *P wave*: Configuration varies
- *PR interval*: Varies with rhythm
- *QRS complex*: 0.10 second
- *T wave*: Configuration varies
- *QT interval*: Varies with rhythm changes

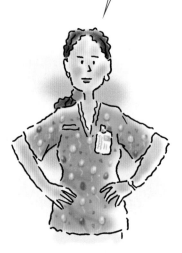

Sick sinus syndrome can promote thrombus formation in the ventricles, leading to thromboembolism.

Recognizing sick sinus syndrome

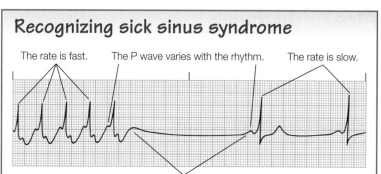

The rate is fast.

The P wave varies with the rhythm.

The rate is slow.

The sinus node doesn't fire, causing a sinus pause.

Atrial arrhythmias

- Are the most common cardiac rhythm disturbances
- Result from impulses originating in areas outside the SA node
- Affect ventricular filling time and diminish the strength of the atrial kick (the contraction that normally provides the ventricles with about 30% of their blood)

Premature atrial contractions

- *Rhythm*: Irregular
- *Rate*: 90 beats/minute
- *P wave*: Abnormal with PAC; some lost in previous T wave
- *PR interval*: 0.16 second
- *QRS complex*: 0.08 second
- *T wave*: Abnormal with some embedded P waves
- *QT interval*: 0.32 second
- *Other*: Noncompensatory pause

(Text continues on page 118.)

Recognizing premature atrial contractions

The rhythm is irregular.   Premature and abnormally shaped P waves occur.

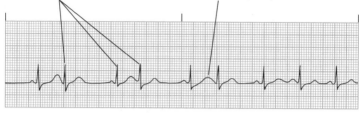

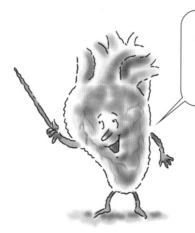

In premature atrial contraction, P waves are sometimes misshapen or lost in the previous T wave.

Atrial arrhythmias *(continued)*

Premature atrial contractions *(continued)*

Distinguishing nonconducted PACs from SA block

- First, look for a nonconducted P wave before, during, or just after the T wave that precedes a pause in rhythm.
- Compare the T waves that precede a pause with the other T waves in the rhythm strip.
  - Look for a distortion in the slope of the T wave or a difference in its height or shape.
  - These distortions may indicate a hidden, nonconducted P wave.
- If a P wave appears in the pause, check to see whether it's premature or whether it occurs earlier than subsequent sinus P waves.
- If the P wave is premature, you can be certain it's a **nonconducted PAC**. (See the shaded area in the top ECG strip to the right.)
- If no P wave appears in the pause or T wave, the rhythm is **SA block**. (See the shaded area on the bottom ECG strip to the right.)

(Text continues on page 120.)

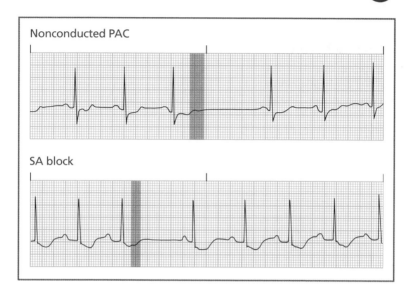

Nonconducted PAC

SA block

Atrial arrhythmias *(continued)*

Atrial tachycardia

- *Rhythm*: Regular
- *Rate*: 210 beats/minute
- *P wave*: Almost hidden in T wave
- *PR interval*: 0.12 second
- *QRS complex*: 0.10 second
- *T wave*: Distorted by P wave
- *QT interval*: 0.20 second

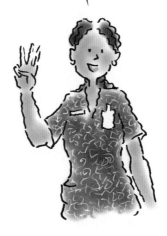

There are three types of atrial tachycardia: atrial tachycardia with block, multifocal atrial tachycardia, and paroxysmal atrial tachycardia.

(Text continues on page 122.)

Recognizing atrial tachycardia

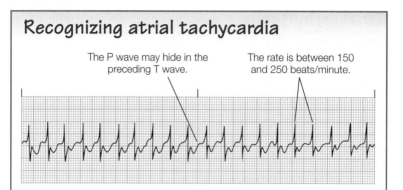

The P wave may hide in the preceding T wave.

The rate is between 150 and 250 beats/minute.

Atrial arrhythmias *(continued)*

Atrial tachycardia *(continued)*

Atrial tachycardia with block

- *Rhythm*: Atrial—regular; ventricular—regular if block is constant, irregular if block is variable
- *Rate*: Atrial—150 to 250 beats/minute, multiple of ventricular rate; ventricular—varies with block
- *P wave*: Slightly abnormal
- *PR interval*: Usually normal; may be hidden
- *QRS complex*: Usually normal
- *T wave*: Usually indistinguishable
- *QT interval*: Indiscernible
- *Other*: More than one P wave for each QRS complex

(Text continues on page 124.)

Recognizing atrial tachycardia with block

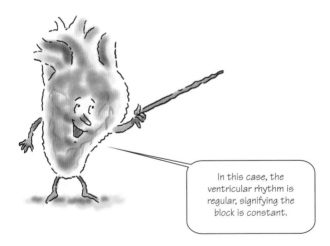

Two P waves occur for each QRS complex.

The ventricular rhythm is regular; the block is constant.

The atrial rhythm is regular.

In this case, the ventricular rhythm is regular, signifying the block is constant.

Atrial arrhythmias *(continued)*
Atrial tachycardia *(continued)*
Multifocal atrial tachycardia (MAT)
- *Rhythm*: Both atrial and ventricular irregular
- *Rate*: Atrial—100 to 250 beats/minute, usually under 160; ventricular —101 to 250 beats/minute
- *P wave*: Configuration varies; must see at least three different P wave shapes
- *PR interval*: Variable
- *QRS complex*: Usually normal
- *T wave*: Usually distorted

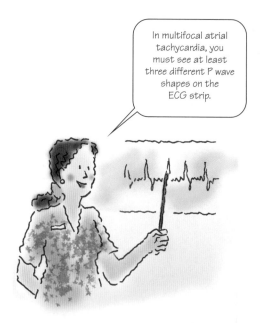

In multifocal atrial tachycardia, you must see at least three different P wave shapes on the ECG strip.

(Text continues on page 126.)

Recognizing multifocal atrial tachycardia

The rhythm is irregular.

The rate is greater than 100 beats/minute.

The configuration of the P wave varies.

Atrial arrhythmias *(continued)*
Atrial tachycardia *(continued)*
Paroxysmal atrial tachycardia (PAT)

- *Rhythm*: Regular
- *Rate*: 140 to 250 beats/minute
- *P wave*: Abnormal; possibly hidden in previous T wave
- *QRS complex*: Possibly aberrantly conducted
- *T wave*: Usually indistinguishable
- *Other*: One P wave for each QRS complex

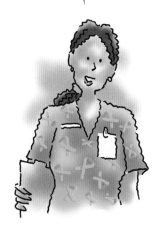

Paroxysmal atrial tachycardia commonly follows frequent premature atrial contractions.

(Text continues on page 128.)

Recognizing paroxysmal atrial tachycardia

The arrhythmia comes on suddenly; in this case, from a PAC.

The rate is 140 to 250 beats/minute

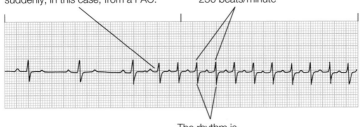

The rhythm is regular.

Atrial arrhythmias *(continued)*

Atrial tachycardia *(continued)*

Distinguishing atrial tachycardia with block from sinus arrhythmia with U waves

● Examine the T wave and the interval from the T wave to the next P wave for evidence of extra P waves. (See the shaded area on the top strip to the right.)

● If extra P waves occur, map them to determine whether they occur at regular intervals (such as with the "normal" P waves).

● In **atrial tachycardia with block**, the P-P intervals are constant.

● Be careful not to mistake a U wave for an extra P wave. (See the shaded area on the bottom strip to the right.)

● The key is to determine if all of the waves occur at regular intervals.

● In **sinus arrhythmia with U waves**, the interval from a U wave to a P wave and a P wave to a U wave won't be constant.

(Text continues on page 130.)

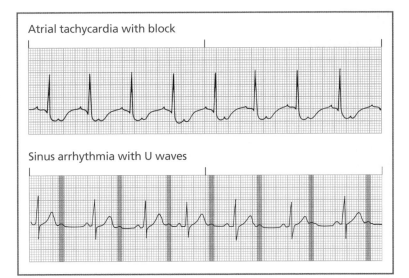

Atrial tachycardia with block

Sinus arrhythmia with U waves

Atrial arrhythmias *(continued)*
Atrial flutter

- *Rhythm*: Atrial—regular; ventricular—irregular
- *Rate*: Atrial—280 beats/minute; ventricular—60 beats/minute
- *P wave*: Classic sawtooth appearance
- *PR interval*: Unmeasurable
- *QRS complex*: 0.08 second
- *T wave*: Unidentifiable
- *Other*: The patient may develop an atrial rhythm that varies between fibrillation and flutter.

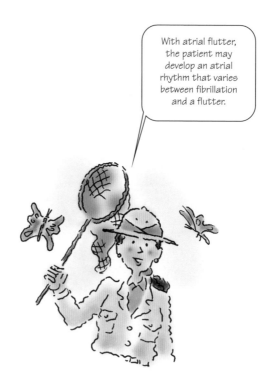

With atrial flutter, the patient may develop an atrial rhythm that varies between fibrillation and a flutter.

(Text continues on page 132.)

Recognizing atrial flutter

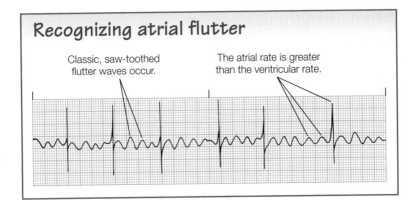

Classic, saw-toothed flutter waves occur.

The atrial rate is greater than the ventricular rate.

Atrial arrhythmias *(continued)*
Atrial fibrillation
- *Rhythm*: Irregularly irregular
- *Rate*: Atrial—indiscernible; ventricular—130 beats/minute
- *P wave*: Absent: replaced by fine fibrillatory waves
- *PR interval*: Indiscernible
- *QRS complex*: 0.08 second
- *T wave*: Indiscernible
- *QT interval*: Unmeasurable

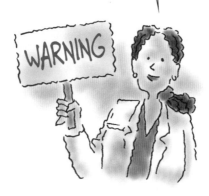

Untreated, atrial fibrillation can lead to cardiovascular collapse, intracardiac thrombus formation, and arterial or pulmonary embolism.

(Text continues on page 134.)

Recognizing atrial fibrillation

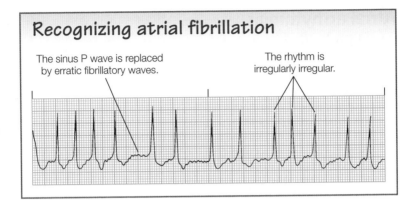

The sinus P wave is replaced by erratic fibrillatory waves.

The rhythm is irregularly irregular.

Atrial arrhythmias *(continued)*
Atrial fibrillation *(continued)*

Distinguishing atrial flutter from atrial fibrillation

- To identify **atrial flutter**, look for characteristic abnormal P waves that produce a sawtooth appearance (referred to as *flutter waves* or *f waves*). (This is best identified in leads I, II, and V_1.)
  - The atrial rhythm should be regular.
  - The F waves can be mapped across the rhythm strip.
  - Some F waves may occur within the QRS or T waves; subsequent F waves are visible and occur on time.
- To identify **atrial fibrillation**, fibrillatory or F waves occur in an irregular pattern, making the atrial rhythm irregular.
- If you identify atrial activity that at times looks like flutter waves and seems to be regular for a short time, and in other places the rhythm strip contains fibrillatory waves, interpret the rhythm as atrial fibrillation.
- Coarse fibrillatory waves may intermittently look similar to the characteristic sawtooth appearance of flutter waves.

(Text continues on page 136.)

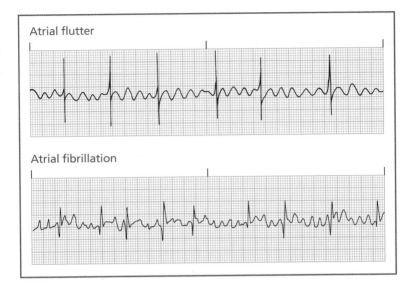

Atrial flutter

Atrial fibrillation

Atrial arrhythmias (continued)
Atrial fibrillation (continued)

Distinguishing atrial fibrillation from MAT

- First, look for discernible P waves before each QRS complex.
- If you can't clearly identify the P waves—and fibrillatory waves, or f waves, appear in the place of P waves—then the rhythm is probably **atrial fibrillation**.
- Next, carefully look at the rhythm, focusing on the R-R intervals; a hallmark of atrial fibrillation is an irregularly irregular rhythm.
- If P waves are present, look at the shape.
  - P waves are present in **MAT**, but the shape of the P wave varies, with at least three different P wave shapes visible in a single rhythm strip.
  - You should be able to see most, if not all, the various P wave shapes repeated.
- Although the atrial and ventricular rhythms are irregular in MAT, the irregularity generally isn't as pronounced as in atrial fibrillation.

(Text continues on page 138.)

Atrial fibrillation

MAT

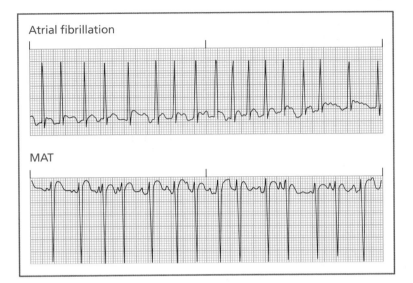

Atrial arrhythmias *(continued)*
Atrial fibrillation *(continued)*
Distinguishing atrial fibrillation from junctional rhythm

- Examine lead I, which provides a clear view of atrial activity.
- Look for fibrillatory or f waves, which appear as a wavy line and indicate fibrillation.
- Chronic **atrial fibrillation** tends to have fine or small f waves and a controlled ventricular rate (below 100 beats/minute).
- To identify **junctional rhythm**, examine lead II.
- If you can find inverted P waves after or within 0.12 second before the QRS complex (see the shaded area in the bottom rhythm strip on the right), then the rhythm is junctional.

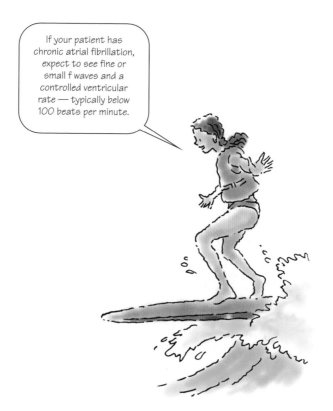

If your patient has chronic atrial fibrillation, expect to see fine or small f waves and a controlled ventricular rate — typically below 100 beats per minute.

Atrial fibrillation

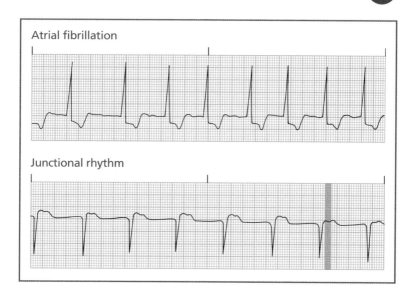

Junctional rhythm

Junctional arrhythmias

● Originate in the AV junction—the area around the AV node and the bundle of His
● Occur when the SA node fails to conduct impulses or when a block in conduction occurs
● Result when pacemaker cells in the AV junction in the middle of the heart produce electrical signals
● Cause the position of the P wave to vary, depending on whether the impulse reaches the atria or ventricles first
– If the atria are depolarized first, the P wave occurs before the QRS complex.
– If the ventricles are depolarized first, the P wave occurs after the QRS complex.
– If the ventricles and atria are depolarized simultaneously, the P wave is hidden in the QRS complex.

(Text continues on page 142.)

Locating the P wave

Atria first

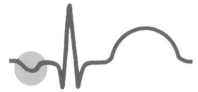

Inverted P wave
before QRS complex

Ventricles first

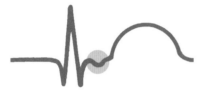

Inverted P wave
after QRS complex

Simultaneous

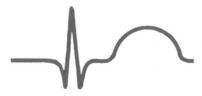

Inverted P wave hidden
in QRS complex

The location of the P wave helps identify the direction of depolarization.

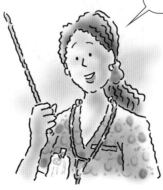

Junctional arrhythmias (continued)
Premature junctional contractions (PJCs)

- *Rhythm*: Atrial and ventricular—irregular
- *Rate*: 100 beats/minute
- *P wave*: Inverted; precedes the QRS complex
- *PR interval*: 0.14 second for the underlying rhythm and 0.06 second for the PJC
- *QRS complex*: 0.06 second
- *T wave*: Normal configuration
- *QT interval*: 0.36 second
- *Other*: Pause after PJC

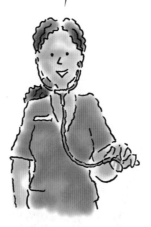

While they're usually nothing to worry about, PJCs can be an early sign of digoxin toxicity.

(Text continues on page 144.)

Recognizing premature junctional contractions

The rhythm is irregular.

The P wave is inverted, with PR interval less than 0.12 second.

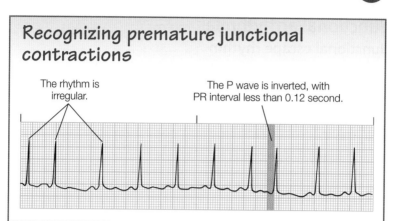

Junctional arrhythmias *(continued)*
Junctional escape rhythm

- *Rhythm*: Regular
- *Rate*: 60 beats/minute
- *P wave*: Inverted; precedes each QRS complex
- *PR interval*: 0.10 second
- *QRS complex*: 0.10 second
- *T wave*: Normal
- *QT interval*: 0.44 second

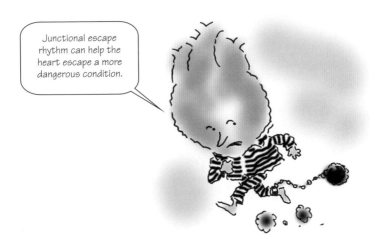

Junctional escape rhythm can help the heart escape a more dangerous condition.

(Text continues on page 146.)

Recognizing junctional escape rhythm

The P wave is inverted.

The rhythm is regular, with a rate of 40 to 60 beats/minute.

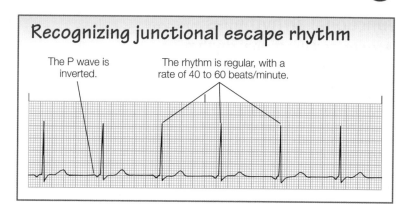

Junctional arrhythmias *(continued)*
Accelerated junctional rhythm

- *Rhythm*: Regular
- *Rate*: 80 beats/minute
- *P wave*: Absent
- *PR interval*: Unmeasurable
- *QRS complex*: 0.10 second
- *T wave*: Normal
- *QT interval*: 0.32 second

(Text continues on page 148.)

Recognizing accelerated junctional rhythm

No P wave appears before the QRS complex.

The rhythm is regular, with a rate between 60 and 100 beats/minute.

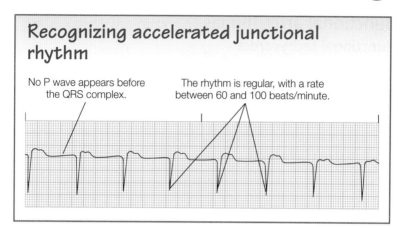

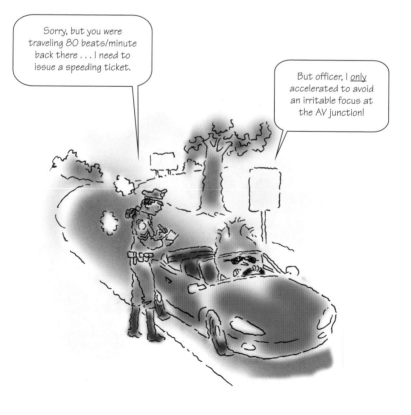

Sorry, but you were traveling 80 beats/minute back there . . . I need to issue a speeding ticket.

But officer, I <u>only</u> accelerated to avoid an irritable focus at the AV junction!

Junctional arrhythmias (continued)
Junctional tachycardia

- *Rhythm*: Regular
- *Rate*: 115 beats/minute
- *P wave*: Inverted; follows the QRS complex
- *PR interval*: Unmeasurable
- *QRS complex*: 0.08 second
- *T wave*: Normal
- *QT interval*: 0.36 second

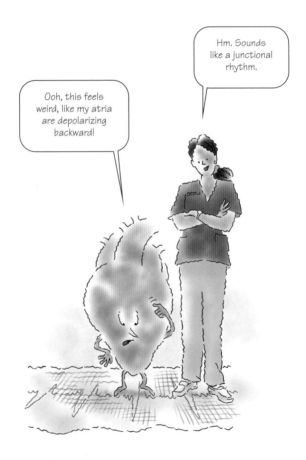

(Text continues on page 150.)

Recognizing junctional tachycardia

The rhythm is regular, with a rate of
100 to 200 beats/minute.

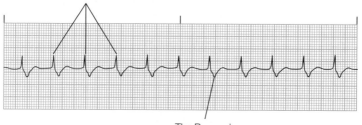

The P wave is
inverted.

Junctional arrhythmias *(continued)*
Wolff-Parkinson-White syndrome

- A common type of preexcitation syndrome
- Commonly occurs in young children and adults ages 20 to 35
- Causes the PR interval to shorten and the QRS complex to lengthen as a result of a delta wave
  - Delta waves occur just before normal ventricular depolarization.
  - Delta waves are produced as a result of the premature depolarization or preexcitation of a portion of the ventricles.
- Considered clinically significant because the accessory pathway—called Kent's bundle—may result in paroxysmal tachyarrhythmias by reentry and rapid conduction mechanisms

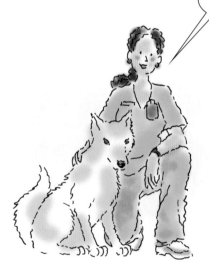

Wolff-Parkinson-White syndrome is typically a congenital rhythm disorder that occurs primarily in young children and in adults ages 20 to 35. Look for the hallmark sign, the delta wave, on ECG.

Recognizing Wolff-Parkinson-White syndrome

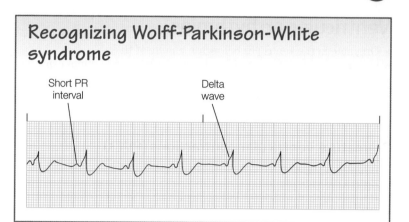

Short PR interval

Delta wave

Ventricular arrhythmias

- Originate in the ventricles below the bundle of His
- Occur when electrical impulses depolarize the myocardium using an abnormal pathway
- Result in a loss of atrial kick, causing cardiac output to decrease by as much as 30%
- Potentially life threatening

Premature ventricular contractions (PVCs)

- *Rhythm*: Irregular
- *Rate*: 120 beats/minute
- *P wave*: Absent with PVC, but present with other QRS complexes
- *PR interval*: 0.12 second in underlying rhythm
- *QRS complex*: Early with bizarre configuration and duration of 0.14 second in PVC; 0.08 second in underlying rhythm
- *T wave*: Normal; opposite direction from QRS complex with PVC
- *QT interval*: 0.28 second with underlying rhythm
- *Other*: Underlying rhythm sinus tachycardia

(Text continues on page 154.)

Recognizing premature ventricular contractions

Premature QRS complex appears wide and bizarre.

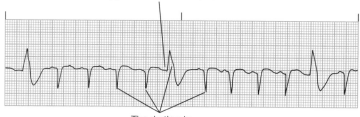

The rhythm is irregular.

Ventricular arrhythmias *(continued)*
Premature ventricular contractions *(continued)*

Paired PVCs
- Consist of two PVCs in a row, as shown in the shaded areas in the top strip on the right
- Also called a ventricular couplet
- Can produce ventricular tachycardia (VT) because the second contraction usually meets refractory tissue
- Considered to be a run of VT when a burst, or salvo, of three or more PVCs occur in a row

Multiform PVCs
- Appear different from each other, as shown in the shaded areas in the bottom strip on the right
- Arise from different sites or from the same site with abnormal conduction
- May indicate severe heart disease or digoxin (Lanoxin) toxicity

(Text continues on page 156.)

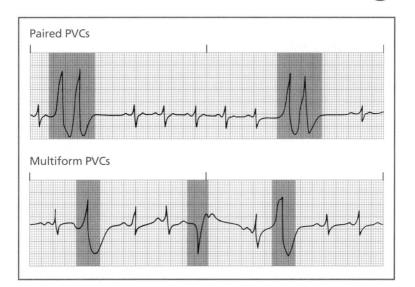

Paired PVCs

Multiform PVCs

Ventricular arrhythmias *(continued)*
Premature ventricular contractions *(continued)*

Bigeminy and trigeminy
- Bigeminy: PVCs that occur every other beat, as shown in the shaded areas in the top strip to the right
- Trigeminy: PVCs that occur every third beat
- May indicate increased ventricular irritability which can result in VT or ventricular fibrillation (VF)

R-on-T phenomenon
- Involves a PVC that occurs so early that it falls on the T wave of the preceding beat, as shown in the shaded areas on the bottom strip to the right
- Can trigger ventricular tachycardia or ventricular fibrillation because the cells haven't had time to fully repolarize

(Text continues on page 158.)

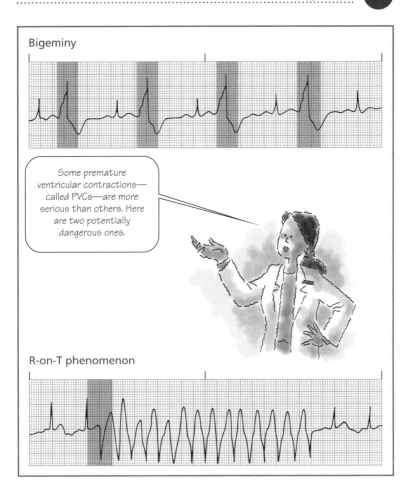

Bigeminy

Some premature ventricular contractions—called PVCs—are more serious than others. Here are two potentially dangerous ones.

R-on-T phenomenon

Ventricular arrhythmias *(continued)*
Idioventricular arrhythmia

- *Rhythm*: Atrial—unmeasurable; ventricular—regular
- *Rate*: Atrial—unmeasurable; ventricular—35 beats/minute
- *P wave*: Absent
- *PR interval*: Unmeasurable
- *QRS complex*: Wide and bizarre
- *T wave*: Deflection opposite to that of the QRS complex
- *QT interval*: 0.60 second

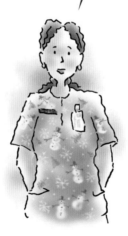

Idioventricular arrhythmia is called the "rhythm of last resort" because it acts to prevent ventricular standstill.

(Text continues on page 160.)

Recognizing idioventricular arrhythmia

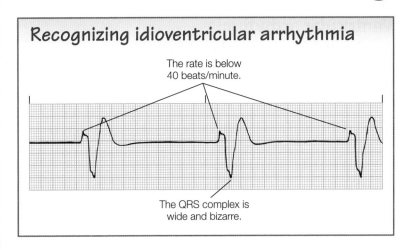

The rate is below 40 beats/minute.

The QRS complex is wide and bizarre.

Ventricular arrhythmias *(continued)*
Accelerated idioventricular arrhythmia

- Has the same characteristics as an idioventricular arrhythmia except that it's faster, as shown in the bottom strip on the right
- Has a rate that's too slow to be called ventricular tachycardia

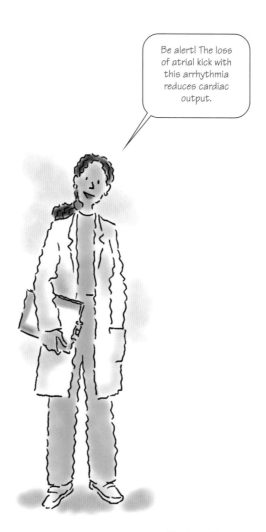

Be alert! The loss of atrial kick with this arrhythmia reduces cardiac output.

(Text continues on page 162.)

Recognizing accelerated idioventricular arrhythmia

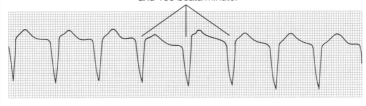

The rate is between 40 and 100 beats/minute.

Ventricular arrhythmias *(continued)*
Ventricular tachycardia

- *Rhythm*: Atrial—unmeasurable; ventricular—usually regular
- *Rate*: Atrial—unmeasurable; ventricular—187 beats/minute
- *P wave*: Absent
- *PR interval*: Unmeasurable
- *QRS complex*: 0.24 second; wide and bizarre
- *T wave*: Opposite direction of QRS complex
- *QT interval*: Unmeasurable
- *Other*: Variations include ventricular flutter and Torsades de pointes

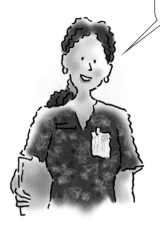

In ventricular tachycardia, or V-tach, three or more PVCs occur in a row and the ventricular rate exceeds 100 beats/minute. It's a significant arrhythmia because of its unpredictability and potential to cause death.

(Text continues on page 164.)

Recognizing ventricular tachycardia

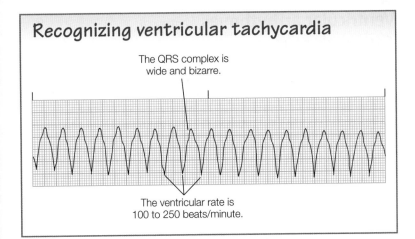

The QRS complex is wide and bizarre.

The ventricular rate is 100 to 250 beats/minute.

Ventricular arrhythmias *(continued)*
Torsades de pointes

- Means "twisting around the points"
- Considered to be a form of polymorphic ventricular tachycardia (VT)
- Has a hallmark appearance of QRS complexes that rotate about the baseline and deflect downward and upward for several beats
- May be paroxysmal, starting and stopping suddenly
- May deteriorate into ventricular fibrillation

(Text continues on page 166.)

Recognizing torsades de pointes

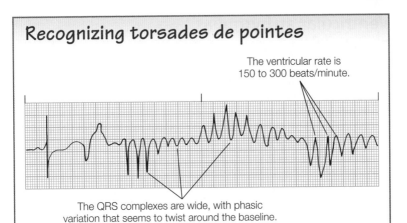

The ventricular rate is 150 to 300 beats/minute.

The QRS complexes are wide, with phasic variation that seems to twist around the baseline.

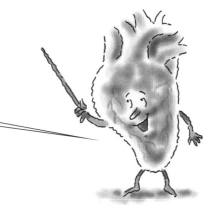

Look for the characteristically wide QRS complexes that rotate about the baseline, deflecting downward and upward for several beats.

Ventricular arrhythmias (continued)
Torsades de pointes (continued)

Distinguishing ventricular flutter from Torsades de pointes

- Consider that **ventricular flutter**:
  - results from the rapid, regular repetitive beating of the ventricles
  - is rarely recognized
  - is produced by a single ventricular focus firing at a rapid rate of 250 to 350 beats/minute
  - has a hallmark appearance of smooth sine waves.
- In contrast, **torsades de pointes**:
  - is a variant form of ventricular tachycardia
  - has a rapid ventricular rate that varies between 250 to 350 beats/minute
  - has QRS complexes that gradually change back and forth, with the amplitude of each successive complex gradually increasing and decreasing
  - produces a rhythm outline commonly described as *spindle-shaped*.

(Text continues on page 168.)

Ventricular flutter

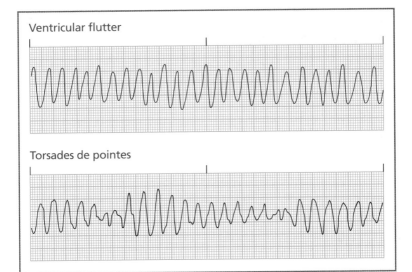

Torsades de pointes

Ventricular arrhythmias *(continued)*
Ventricular fibrillation

- *Rhythm*: Chaotic
- *Rate*: Indiscernible
- *P wave*: Absent
- *R interval*: Unmeasurable
- *QRS complex*: Indiscernible
- *T wave*: Indiscernible
- *QT interval*: Indiscernible
- *Other*: Waveform is a wavy line

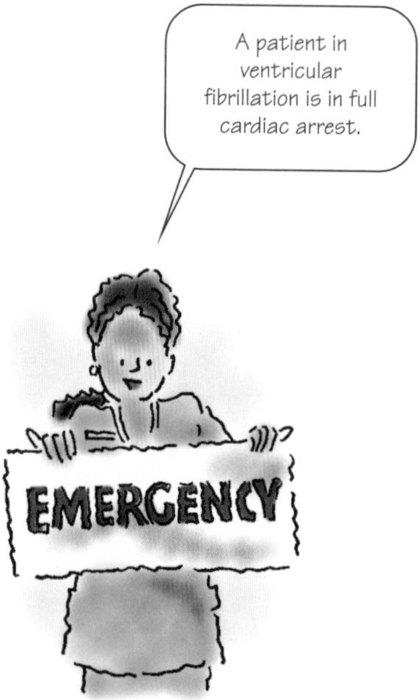

Recognizing ventricular fibrillation

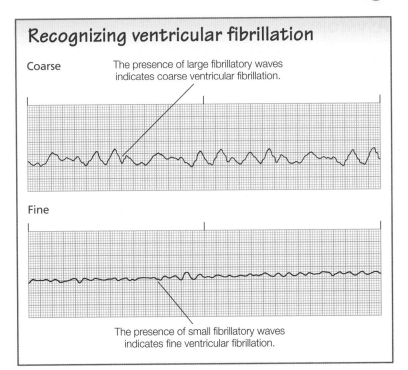

Coarse

The presence of large fibrillatory waves indicates coarse ventricular fibrillation.

Fine

The presence of small fibrillatory waves indicates fine ventricular fibrillation.

Asystole

- Involves the absence of electrical activity in the ventricles
- *Rhythm*: Atrial—indiscernible; ventricular—absent
- *Rate*: Atrial—indiscernible; ventricular—absent
- *P wave*: May be present
- *PR interval*: Unmeasurable
- *QRS complex*: Absent or occasional escape beats
- *T wave*: Absent
- *QT interval*: Unmeasurable
- *Other*: On a rhythm strip, asystole looks like a nearly flat line (except for changes caused by chest compressions during CPR). In a patient with a pacemaker, pacer spikes may be evident on the strip but no P wave or QRS complex occurs in response to the stimulus.

Recognizing asystole

The absence of electrical activity in the ventricles results in a nearly flat line.

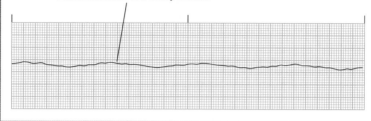

Also called ventricular standstill, asystole looks like a nearly flat line on a rhythm strip, except for changes caused by chest compression during CPR.

Pulseless electrical activity

● *Rhythm*: Atrial—same as the underlying rhythm; ventricular—same as the underlying rhythm; both become irregular as the rate slows
● *Rate*: Atrial—reflects the underlying rhythm; ventricular—reflects the underlying rhythm; eventually both decrease
● *P wave*: Same as the underlying rhythm; gradually flattens and then disappears
● *PR interval*: Same as the underlying rhythm; eventually disappears as the P wave disappears
● *QRS complex*: Same as the underlying rhythm; becomes progressively wider
● *T wave*: Same as the underlying rhythm; eventually becomes indiscernible
● *QT interval*: Same as the underlying rhythm; eventually becomes indiscernible
● *Other*: Usually becomes a flat line indicating asystole within several minutes

Recognizing pulseless electrical activity

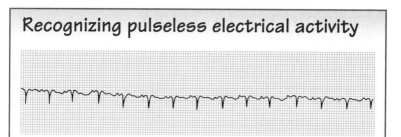

Atrioventricular (AV) block

- Results from an interruption in the conduction of impulses between the atria and ventricles
- Can be total or partial
- Can delay conduction
- Can occur at the AV node, bundle of His, or bundle branches

First-degree AV block

- *Rhythm*: Regular
- *Rate*: 75 beats/minute
- *P wave*: Normal
- *PR interval*: 0.32 second
- *QRS complex*: 0.08 second
- *T wave*: Normal
- *QT interval*: 0.40 second

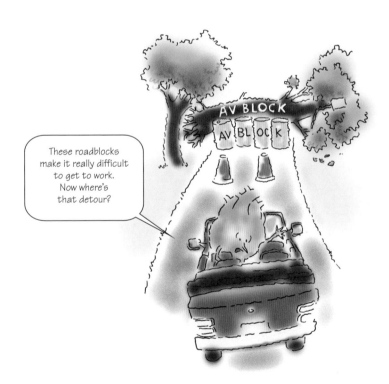

(Text continues on page 176.)

Recognizing first-degree AV block

The PR interval is greater than 0.20 second.

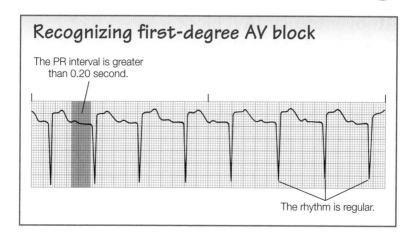

The rhythm is regular.

Atrioventricular (AV) block *(continued)*
Type I second-degree AV block

- Also known as Wenckebach or Mobitz I
- *Rhythm*: Atrial—regular; ventricular—irregular
- *Rate*: Atrial—80 beats/minute; ventricular—50 beats/minute
- *P wave*: Normal
- *PR interval*: Progressively prolonged
- *QRS complex*: 0.08 second
- *T wave*: Normal
- *QT interval*: 0.46 second
- *Other*: Wenckebach pattern of grouped beats

> Type I second-degree AV block may occur normally in an otherwise healthy person.

(Text continues on page 178.)

Recognizing type I second-degree AV block

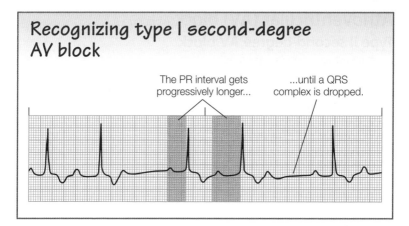

The PR interval gets progressively longer...

...until a QRS complex is dropped.

Atrioventricular (AV) block *(continued)*
Type II second-degree AV block

- Also known as Mobitz II block
- *Rhythm*: Atrial—regular; ventricular—irregular
- *Rate*: Atrial—60 beats/minute; ventricular—50 beats/minute
- *P wave*: Normal
- *PR interval*: 0.28 second
- *QRS complex*: 0.10 second
- *T wave*: Normal
- *QT interval*: 0.60 second

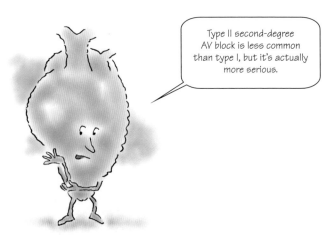

Type II second-degree AV block is less common than type I, but it's actually more serious.

(Text continues on page 180.)

Recognizing type II second-degree AV block

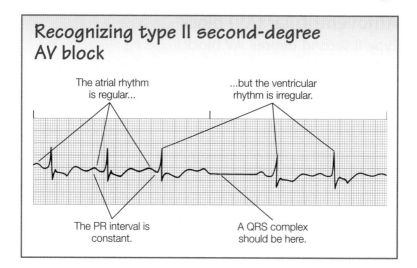

The atrial rhythm is regular...

...but the ventricular rhythm is irregular.

The PR interval is constant.

A QRS complex should be here.

Atrioventricular (AV) block *(continued)*
Type II second-degree AV block *(continued)*

Distinguishing nonconducted PACs from type II second-degree AV block

● An isolated P wave that doesn't conduct through to the ventricle (a P wave without a QRS complex following it) may occur with a non-conducted premature PAC or it may indicate a type II second-degree AV block.

● If the P-P interval, including the extra P wave, isn't constant, it's a **nonconducted PAC** (as shown by the top strip on the right).

● If the P-P interval, including the extra P wave, is constant, it's **type II second degree AV block** (as shown by the bottom strip on the right).

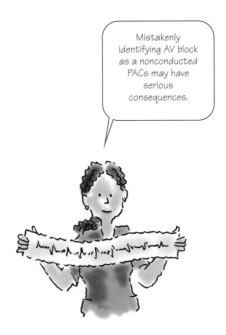

> Mistakenly identifying AV block as a nonconducted PACs may have serious consequences.

(Text continues on page 182.)

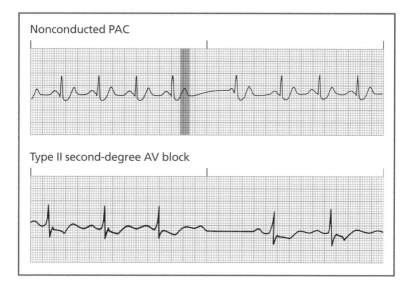

Nonconducted PAC

Type II second-degree AV block

Atrioventricular (AV) block *(continued)*

Third-degree AV block

- Also called complete heart block
- *Rhythm*: Regular
- *Rate*: Atrial—90 beats/minute; ventricular—30 beats/minute
- *P wave*: Normal
- *PR interval*: Variable
- *QRS complex*: 0.16 second
- *T wave*: Normal
- *QT interval*: 0.56 second

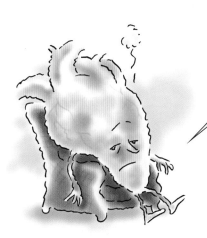

> This arrhythmia is characterized by the complete absence of impulse conduction between my atria and ventricula. Treatment and prognosis vary depending on the anatomic level of the block.

(Text continues on page 184.)

Recognizing third-degree AV block

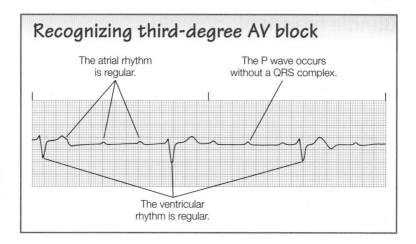

The atrial rhythm is regular.

The P wave occurs without a QRS complex.

The ventricular rhythm is regular.

Bundle branch block (BBB)

- Results when the left or right bundle branch fails to conduct impulses
- Called a *hemiblock* or *fascicular block* when the BBB occurs low in the left bundle branch
- Requires the impulse to travel down the unaffected bundle branch and then from one myocardial cell to the next to depolarize the ventricle
- Causes a widened QRS complex as a result of the prolonged depolarization
- Identified by a QRS complex greater than 0.12 second

Right bundle branch block (RBBB)

- Revealed in lead V_1 by a small r wave (showing left ventricular depolarization) followed by a large R wave (confirming right ventricular depolarization)
- Revealed in lead V_6 by a widened S wave and upright T wave

(Text continues on page 186.)

Recognizing right bundle branch block

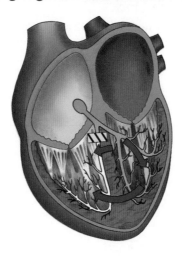

Lead V₁

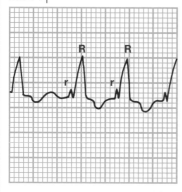

Lead V₆

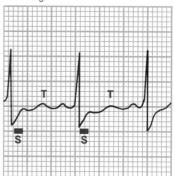

Bundle branch block (BBB) *(continued)*
Left bundle branch block

- Revealed in lead V_1 by no R wave and a wide, large QS wave
- Revealed in lead V_6 by slurred R waves and inverted T waves

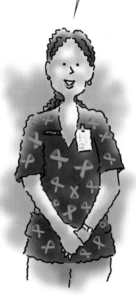

Frequently, bundle branch block is monitored only to detect whether it progresses to a more complete block.

(Text continues on page 188.)

Recognizing left bundle branch block

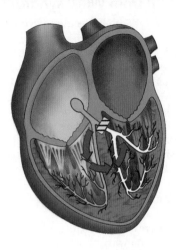

Lead V$_1$

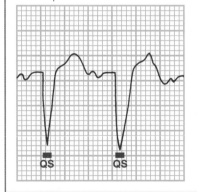

QS   QS

Lead V$_6$

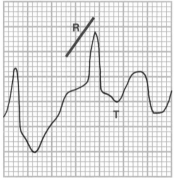

R

T

Bundle branch block (BBB) (continued)
Distinguishing BBB from WPW syndrome

- Carefully examine the QRS complex, noting which part of the complex is widened.
- A **BBB** involves a defective conduction of the electrical impulses through the right or left bundle branch from the bundle of His to the Purkinje network, causing a right or left block.
  - This conduction disturbance results in an overall increase in QRS duration, or widening of the last part of the QRS complex, while the initial part of the QRS complex appears normal.
  - The change is consistent in all leads.
  - PR intervals are normal unless an AV conduction defect is causing a prolonged PR interval.
- In **WPW syndrome**, a delta wave occurs at the beginning of the QRS complex, usually causing a distinctive slurring or hump on its initial slope.
  - Delta waves are not present in BBB.
  - On a 12-lead ECG, delta waves are most pronounced in the leads "looking at" the part of the heart where the accessory pathway is located.
  - The delta wave shortens the PR interval in WPW syndrome.

Bundle branch block

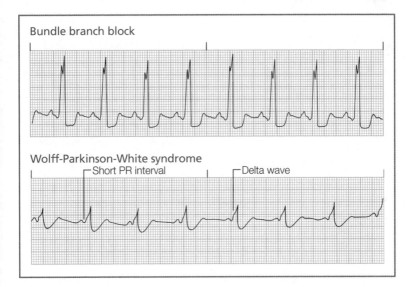

Wolff-Parkinson-White syndrome

┌─Short PR interval   ┌─Delta wave

4

Disorder-related ECG changes

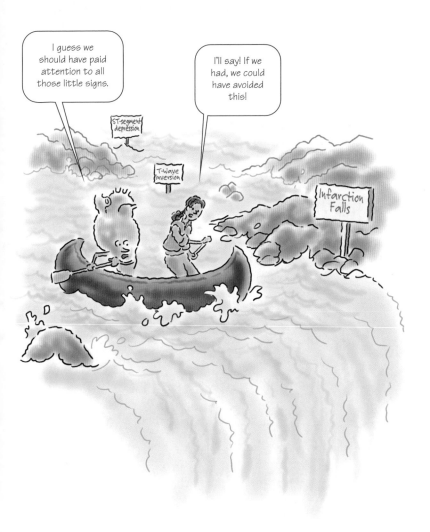

Angina

- Classified as an acute coronary syndrome
- Occurs as one of two types:
  - Stable angina: Occurs in a predictable, repetitive pattern
  - Unstable angina: Commonly signals an MI
- Results when the myocardium demands more oxygen than the coronary arteries can deliver
- Produces episodic pain, usually lasting 2 to 10 minutes; pain persisting as long as 30 minutes suggests myocardial infarction (MI) rather than angina
- Produces specific ECG changes:
  - Peaked T waves
  - Flattened T waves
  - T-wave inversion
  - ST-segment depression with T-wave inversion
  - T-segment depression without T-wave inversion

ECG changes in angina

Peaked T wave

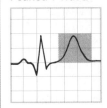

Flattened T wave

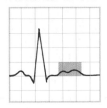

T-wave inversion

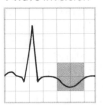

ST-segment depression with T-wave inversion

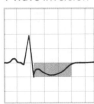

ST-segment depression without T-wave inversion

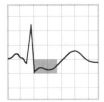

Prinzmetal's angina

- A relatively uncommon form of unstable angina
- Results from a focal episodic spasm of a coronary artery
- Almost always causes pain at rest as opposed to following activity
- *Rhythm*: Atrial and ventricular are normal
- *Rate*: Atrial and ventricular are within normal limits
- *P wave*: Normal size and configuration
- *PR interval*: Normal
- *QRS complex*: Normal
- *ST-segment*: Elevations in leads monitoring the area of coronary artery spasm; elevations occur during chest pain and resolve when the pain subsides
- *T waves*: Usually of normal size and configuration
- *QT interval*: Normal

ECG changes in Prinzmetal's angina

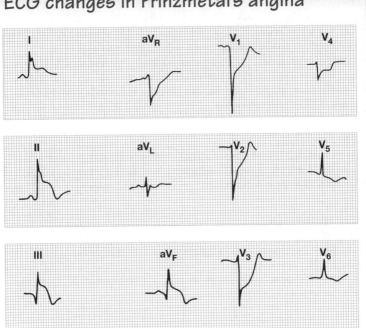

Myocardial infarction

- Categorized as an acute coronary syndrome
- Occurs when reduced blood flow through one or more coronary arteries causes myocardial ischemia, injury, and necrosis
- Usually causes damage in the left ventricle, but the location can vary depending on the coronary artery affected
- Causes three pathologic changes that are reflected on an ECG: ischemia, injury, and infarction

Ischemia

- The first stage
- Indicates that blood flow is out of balance with oxygen demand
- Can be resolved by improving blood flow or reducing oxygen needs
- Causes ST-segment depression or T-wave inversion

Injury

- The second stage
- Indicates injury
- Occurs when the ischemia is prolonged enough to damage an area of the heart
- Causes ST-segment elevation, usually in two or more contiguous leads, as well as T-wave inversion

(Text continues on page 198.)

Recognizing myocardial ischemia and injury

Ischemia

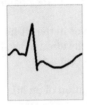

- T-wave inversion
- ST-depression

Injury

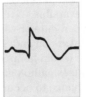

- ST-segment elevation
- T-wave inversion

Myocardial infarction (continued)

Infarction

- The third stage
- Occurs when myocardial cells die
- Results in the development of scar tissue to replace dead tissue, making the damage irreversible
- May produce hyperacute or very tall T waves in the earliest stage
- Causes T-wave inversion and ST-segment elevation in the leads facing the area of damage within hours of the infarction
- Eventually produces pathologic Q waves
    - This the last change to occur in the evolution of an MI.
    - It is the only permanent ECG evidence of myocardial necrosis.

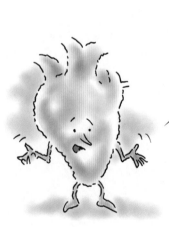

Pathologic Q waves are the last change to occur in the evolution of an MI. They're also the only permanent ECG evidence of myocardial tissue death. Who knew?

(Text continues on page 200.)

Recognizing myocardial infarction

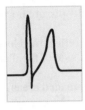

- Hyperacute T waves
(earliest stage)

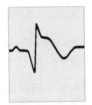

- ST-segment elevation
- T-wave inversion
- Pathologic Q waves
  - in 90% of ST-segment elevation MI
  - in 25% non–ST-segment elevation MI

Myocardial infarction *(continued)*
Reciprocal changes in MI

- Ischemia, injury, and infarction—the three I's of MI—disrupt normal depolarization.
- Characteristic ECG changes arise in the leads that reflect the electrical activity in the damaged areas (shown on the right side of the illustration to the right).
- Reciprocal changes appear in leads opposite the damaged areas (shown on the left side of the illustration to the right).

(Text continues on page 202.)

Understanding reciprocal changes in MI

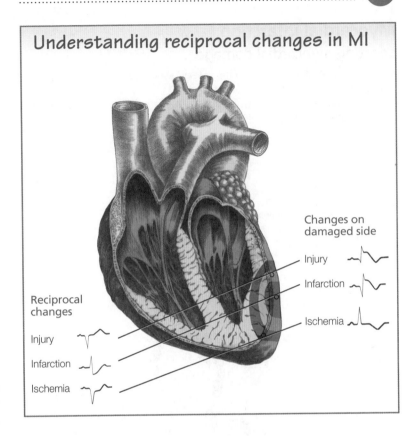

Changes on damaged side

Injury

Infarction

Ischemia

Reciprocal changes

Injury

Infarction

Ischemia

Myocardial infarction (continued)
Locating myocardial damage

- The leads showing changes characteristic of an MI will vary, depending on the area of infarction.
- Identifying the leads showing changes helps pinpoint the heart wall affected and the artery involved.

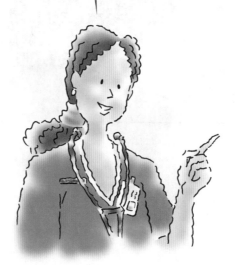

The location of an MI is a critical factor in determining the most appropriate treatment and predicting probable complications.

(Text continues on page 204.)

Locating myocardial damage

Wall affected	Leads	Artery involved	Reciprocal changes
Anterior	V_2, V_3, V_4	Left coronary artery, left anterior descending (LAD)	II, III, aV_F
Anterolateral	I, aV_L, V_3, V_4, V_5, V_6	LAD and diagonal branches, circumflex and marginal branches	II, III, aV_F
Anteroseptal	V_1, V_2, V_3, V_4	LAD	None
Inferior	II, III, aV_F	Right coronary artery (RCA)	I, aV_L
Lateral	I, aV_L, V_5, V_6	Circumflex branch of left coronary artery	II, III, aV_F
Posterior	V_8, V_9	RCA or circumflex	V_1, V_2, V_3, V_4 (R greater than S in V_1 and V_2, ST-segment depression, elevated T wave)
Right ventricular	V_{4R}, V_{5R}, V_{6R}	RCA	None

Myocardial infarction *(continued)*
Anterior-wall MI

- Causes characteristic ECG changes in leads V_2 to V_4
- Precordial leads show:
  - poor R-wave progression
  - ST-segment elevation
  - T-wave inversion.
- Reciprocal changes—appearing in inferior leads I, III, and aV_F—include:
  - initially tall R waves
  - depressed ST segments.

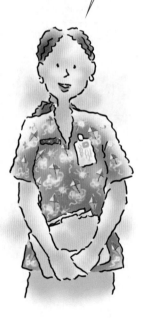

When the left anterior descending artery becomes occluded, an anterior-wall MI occurs.

(Text continues on page 206.)

Recognizing an anterior-wall MI

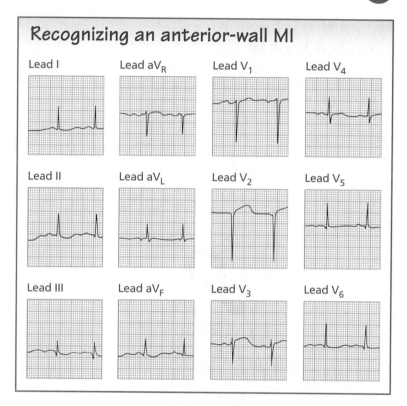

Lead I   Lead aV$_R$ Lead V$_1$ Lead V$_4$

Lead II   Lead aV$_L$ Lead V$_2$ Lead V$_5$

Lead III   Lead aV$_F$ Lead V$_3$ Lead V$_6$

Myocardial infarction *(continued)*
Anteroseptal-wall MI

- Causes loss of the R wave in leads V_1 and V_2
- Also causes ST-segment elevation in leads V_1 to V_4

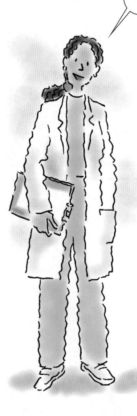

Because the left anterior descending artery also supplies blood to the ventricular septum, a septal-wall MI typically accompanies an anterior-wall MI.

(Text continues on page 208.)

Recognizing an anteroseptal-wall MI

Myocardial infarction *(continued)*
Inferior-wall MI

- Causes the following changes in leads II, III, and aV_F:
  - T-wave inversion
  - ST-segment elevation
  - pathologic Q waves
- Causes a reciprocal change of slight ST-segment depression in leads I and aV_L

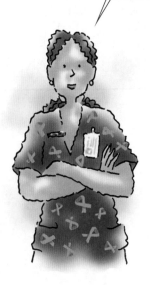

An inferior-wall MI is also called a diaphragmatic MI. That's because the heart's inferior wall lies over the diaphragm.

(Text continues on page 210.)

Recognizing an inferior-wall MI

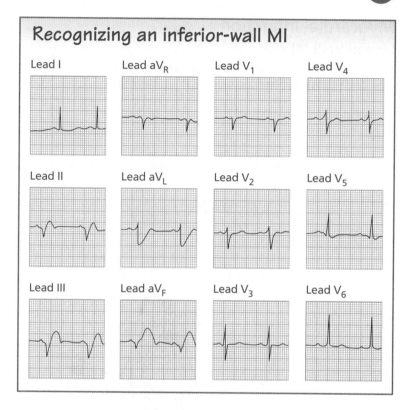

Lead I Lead aV_R Lead V_1 Lead V_4

Lead II Lead aV_L Lead V_2 Lead V_5

Lead III Lead aV_F Lead V_3 Lead V_6

Myocardial infarction *(continued)*
Lateral-wall MI

- Shows ST-segment elevation in leads I, aV_L, V_5, and V_6.
- Displays reciprocal changes in leads II, III, and aV_F.

A lateral-wall MI is usually caused by a blockage in the left circumflex artery.

(Text continues on page 212.)

Recognizing a lateral-wall MI

Myocardial infarction *(continued)*
Right-ventricular-wall MI

- Causes ST-segment elevation in the right precordial leads V_{4R}, V_{5R}, and V_{6R}.
- May also produce pathologic Q waves in leads V_{4R}, V_{5R}, and V_{6R}.

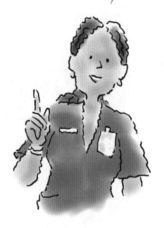

Be on the lookout. A right ventricular MI can lead to right-sided heart failure or right-sided heart block.

Recognizing a right-ventricular-wall MI

Left-side leads   Right-side leads

Pericarditis

- Changes vary according to stage of illness
- **Stage 1** changes reflect inflammation and include:
  - diffuse ST-segment elevations of 1 to 2 mm in most limb leads and most precordial leads
  - upright T-waves in most leads
  - ST-segment and T-wave changes in leads I, II, III, aV_R, aV_F, and V_2 through V_6.
- **Stage 2** changes reflect resolving pericarditis and include:
  - resolution of ST-segment elevation
  - widespread T-wave inversion.

(Text continues on page 216.)

Recognizing pericarditis

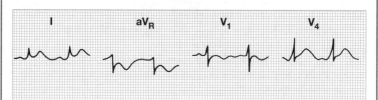

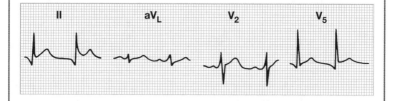

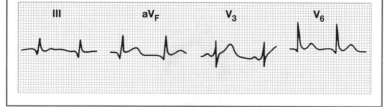

Pericarditis (continued)

Distinguishing MI from acute pericarditis

● Although both MI and acute pericarditis cause ST-segment elevation, the ST segment and T wave appear different on an MI waveform compared to those on a pericarditis waveform.

● In pericarditis, several leads will show ST-segment and T-wave changes; in MI, only those leads reflecting the area of infarction will show the characteristic changes.

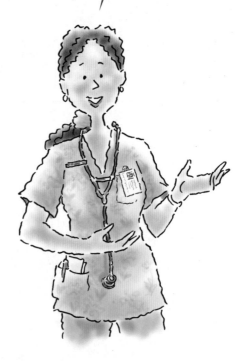

Because pericarditis usually affects the entire myocardial surface, ST segments are usually elevated in most—if not all—leads.

Comparing MI with acute pericarditis

Acute pericarditis

MI

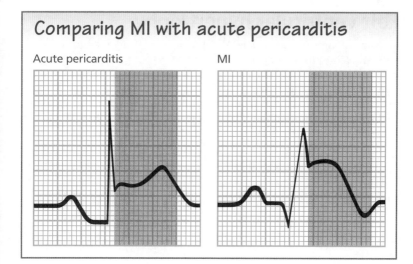

Left ventricular hypertrophy

● Causes a large S wave in lead V_1 (shown in the shaded area on the strip labeled V_1 to the right)
● Causes a large R wave in lead V_5 (shown in the shaded area on the strip labeled V_5 to the right)
● Can be confirmed if the depth (in mm) of the S wave in lead V_1 added to the height (in mm) of the R wave in lead V_6 is greater than 35 mm

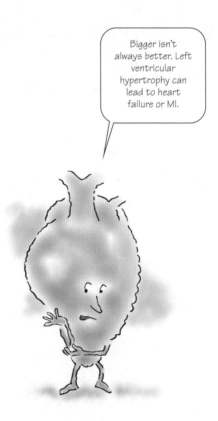

Bigger isn't always better. Left ventricular hypertrophy can lead to heart failure or MI.

Recognizing left ventricular hypertrophy

Lead V₁

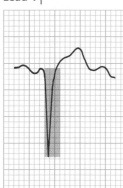

Lead V₅

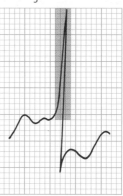

5

Drug- and electrolyte-related ECG changes

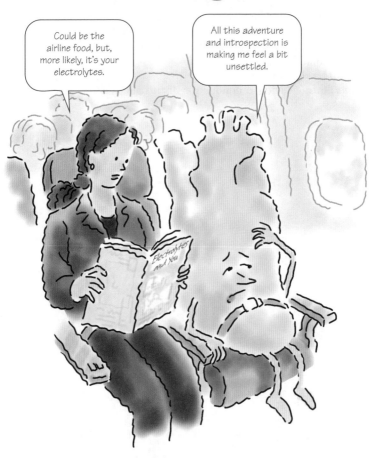

Electrolyte imbalances

- Potassium and calcium play a key role in the heart's electrical activity.
- Imbalances in electrolytes frequently produce distinctive rhythm changes on ECGs.

Hyperkalemia

- *Rhythm*: Regular (both atrial and ventricular)
- *Rate*: Within normal limits (both atrial and ventricular)
- *P wave*: Low amplitude in mild hyperkalemia; wide and flattened in moderate hyperkalemia; may be indiscernible in severe hyperkalemia
- *PR interval*: Normal or prolonged; not measurable if P wave is indiscernible
- *QRS complex*: Widened due to prolonged ventricular depolarization
- *ST segment*: May be elevated in severe hyperkalemia
- *T wave*: Tall and peaked—the classic and most striking feature of hyperkalemia
- *QT interval*: Shortened
- *Other*: Intraventricular conduction disturbances commonly occur

(Text continues on page 224.)

Recognizing the effects of hyperkalemia

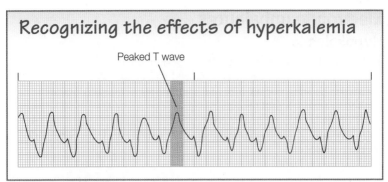

Peaked T wave

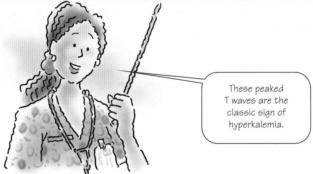

These peaked T waves are the classic sign of hyperkalemia.

Electrolyte imbalances *(continued)*
Hypokalemia

- *Rhythm*: Regular (both atrial and ventricular)
- *Rate*: Within normal limits (both atrial and ventricular)
- *P wave*: Usually normal size and configuration but may become peaked in severe hypokalemia
- *PR interval*: May be prolonged
- *QRS complex*: Within normal limits or possibly widened; prolonged in severe hypokalemia
- *ST segment*: Depressed
- *T wave*: Decreased amplitude; becomes flat as potassium level drops
  - In severe hypokalemia, T wave flattens completely and may become inverted.
  - T wave may also infuse with an increasingly prominent U wave.
- *QT interval*: Usually indiscernible as the T wave flattens
- *Other*: Amplitude of the U wave is increased, becoming more prominent as hypokalemia worsens and it fuses with the T wave.

(Text continues on page 226.)

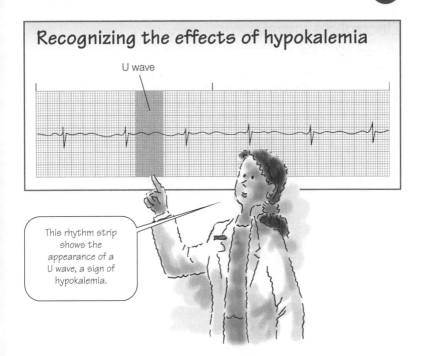

Recognizing the effects of hypokalemia

U wave

This rhythm strip shows the appearance of a U wave, a sign of hypokalemia.

Electrolyte imbalances *(continued)*

Hypercalcemia

- *Rhythm*: Regular (both atrial and ventricular)
- *Rate*: Within normal limits (both atrial and ventricular) but bradycardia can occur
- *P wave*: Normal size and configuration
- *PR interval*: May be prolonged
- *QRS complex*: Within normal limits, but may be prolonged
- *ST segment*: Shortened
- *T wave*: Normal size and configuration; may be depressed
- *QT interval*: Shortened

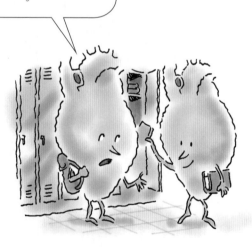

(Text continues on page 228.)

Recognizing the effects of hypercalcemia

Shortened QT interval

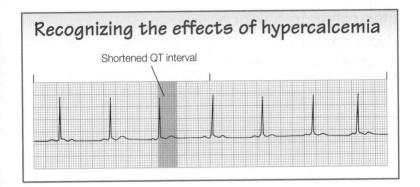

Electrolyte imbalances *(continued)*
Hypocalcemia

- *Rhythm*: Regular (both atrial and ventricular)
- *Rate*: Within normal limits (both atrial and ventricular)
- *P wave*: Normal size and configuration
- *PR interval*: Within normal limits
- *QRS complex*: Within normal limits
- *ST segment*: Prolonged
- *T wave*: Normal size and configuration, but may become flat or inverted
- *QT interval*: Prolonged

Recognizing the effects of hypocalcemia

Prolonged QT interval

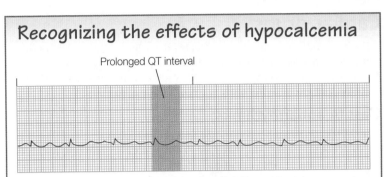

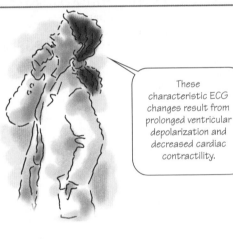

These characteristic ECG changes result from prolonged ventricular depolarization and decreased cardiac contractility.

Cardiac drugs

- Because antiarrhythmics can affect the cardiac cell's action potential, characteristic ECG changes can occur.
- Drugs such as digoxin (Lanoxin) may also exhibit characteristic ECG patterns that can provide early warnings of drug toxicity.

Class IA antiarrhythmics

- Includes drugs such as quinidine and procainamide
- Block sodium influx during phase 0 of the action potential, which depresses the rate of depolarization
- Prolong repolarization and the duration of the action potential
- Lengthen the refractory period
- Decrease contractility
- *QRS complex*: Slightly widened; increased widening is an early sign of toxicity
- *T wave*: May be flattened or inverted
- *QT interval*: Prolonged
- *U wave*: May be present

(Text continues on page 232.)

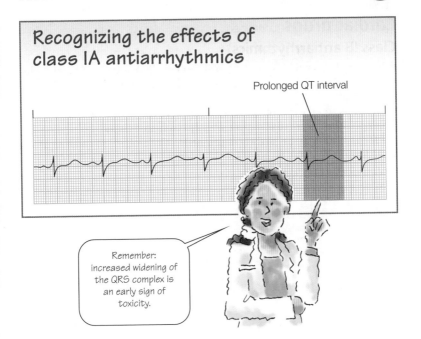

Recognizing the effects of class IA antiarrhythmics

Prolonged QT interval

Remember: increased widening of the QRS complex is an early sign of toxicity.

Cardiac drugs *(continued)*
Class IB antiarrhythmics

- Include drugs such as phenytoin (Dilantin), lidocaine, and mexiletine
- Block sodium influx during phase 0, which depresses the role of depolarization
- Shortens repolarization and the duration of the action potential
- Suppresses ventricular automaticity in ischemic tissue
- *PR interval*: May be slightly shortened
- *QRS complex*: May be slightly widened
- *QT interval*: Shortened

(Text continues on page 234.)

Recognizing the effects of class IB antiarrhythmics

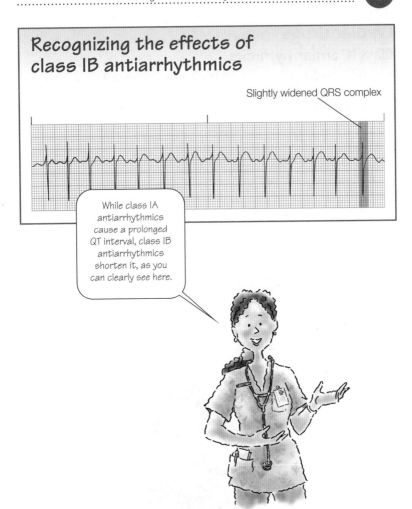

Slightly widened QRS complex

While class IA antiarrhythmics cause a prolonged QT interval, class IB antiarrhythmics shorten it, as you can clearly see here.

Cardiac drugs *(continued)*
Class IC antiarrhythmics

- Includes such drugs as flecainide (Tambocor), propafenone (Rythmol), and moricizine
- Block sodium influx during phase 0, which depresses the rate of depolarization
- Exert no effect on repolarization or the duration of the action potential
- *PR interval*: Prolonged
- *QRS complex*: Prolonged
- *QT interval*: Prolonged

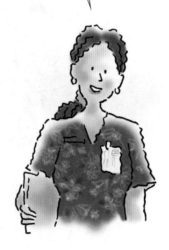

Class IC antiarrhythmics are usually reserved for refractory arrhythmias because they may cause or worsen arrhythmias.

(Text continues on page 236.)

Recognizing the effects of class IC antiarrhythmics

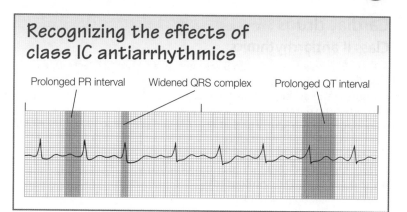

Prolonged PR interval   Widened QRS complex   Prolonged QT interval

Cardiac drugs *(continued)*
Class II antiarrhythmics
- Include beta-adrenergic blockers such as acebutolol (Sectral), esmolol (Brevibloc), and propranolol (Inderal)
- Depress sinoatrial node automaticity
- Shorten the duration of the action potential
- Increase the refractory period of atrial and atrioventricular junctional tissues, which slows conduction
- Inhibit sympathetic activity
- *Rate*: Decreased (both atrial and ventricular)
- *PR interval*: Slightly prolonged
- *QT interval*: Slightly shortened

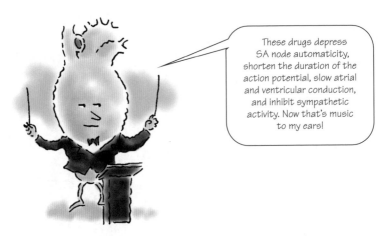

These drugs depress SA node automaticity, shorten the duration of the action potential, slow atrial and ventricular conduction, and inhibit sympathetic activity. Now that's music to my ears!

(Text continues on page 238.)

Recognizing the effects of class II antiarrhythmics

Slightly prolonged PR interval

Slightly shortened QT interval

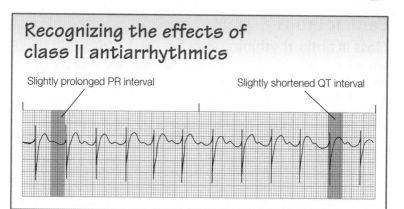

Cardiac drugs *(continued)*
Class III antiarrhythmics

- Include drugs such as amiodarone (Cordarone), sotalol (Betapace), and ibutilide (Corvert)
- Block potassium movement during phase 3
- Increase the duration of the action potential
- Prolong the effective refractory period
- *PR interval*: Prolonged
- *QRS complex*: Widened
- *QT interval*: Prolonged

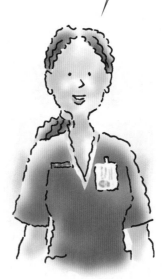

Class III antiarrhythmics are called potassium channel blockers because they block the movement of potassium during phase 3 of the action potential.

(Text continues on page 240.)

Recognizing the effects of class III antiarrhythmics

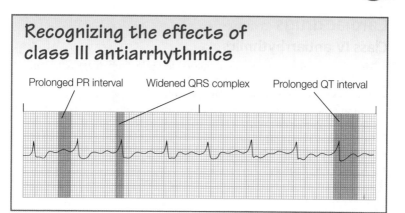

Prolonged PR interval   Widened QRS complex   Prolonged QT interval

Cardiac drugs *(continued)*
Class IV antiarrhythmics

- Also called calcium channel blockers; include such drugs as verapamil (Calan) and diltiazem (Cardizem)
- Block calcium movement during phase 2
- Prolong the conduction time and increase the refractory period in the atrioventricular node
- Decrease contractility
- *Rate*: Decreased (both atrial and ventricular)
- *PR interval*: Prolonged

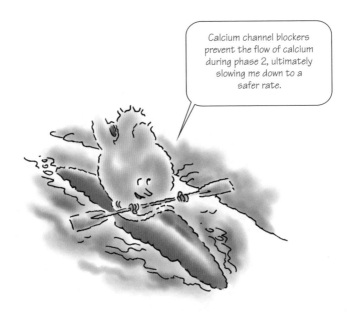

Calcium channel blockers prevent the flow of calcium during phase 2, ultimately slowing me down to a safer rate.

(Text continues on page 242.)

Recognizing the effects of class IV antiarrhythmics

Prolonged PR interval

Cardiac drugs *(continued)*

Digoxin

- Has a very narrow window of therapeutic effectiveness
- May cause numerous arrhythmias at toxic levels, including paroxysmal atrial tachycardia with block, AV block, atrial and junctional tachyarrhythmias, and ventricular arrhythmias
- *Rate*: Decreased (both atrial and ventricular)
- *PR interval*: Shortened
- *ST segment*: Shortened and depressed; sagging (scooping or sloping) of the segment is characteristic
- *T wave*: Decreased
- *QT interval*: Shortened due to the shortened ST segment

(Text continues on page 244.)

Recognizing the effects of digoxin

ST-segment depression in the opposite
direction of the QRS deflection

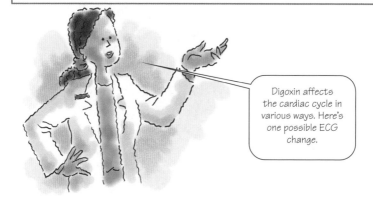

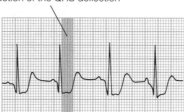

Digoxin affects
the cardiac cycle in
various ways. Here's
one possible ECG
change.

Cardiac drugs *(continued)*

Adenosine

- Affects conduction through the atrioventricular node
- Commonly causes an asystolic pause that lasts a few seconds at the time of conversion
- *Rate*: Varies; initially tachycardic and then becomes normal
- *PR interval*: Difficult to determine initially; later becomes normal or, occasionally, exhibits a first-degree block
- *QT interval*: Shortened because of the increased heart rate; becomes normal when the heart rate slows

Recognizing the effects of adenosine

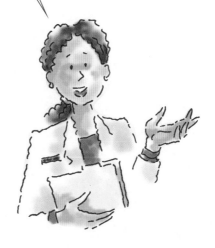

Because adenosine affects conduction through the AV node, it may lead to the ECG changes shown here.

6

Pacemakers and the ECG

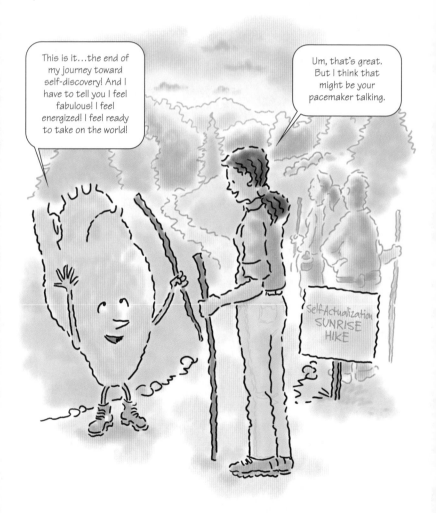

Pacemakers

- Artificial devices that electronically stimulate the myocardium to depolarize, initiating mechanical contractions
- Use pacing leads that can be unipolar (one electrode) or bipolar (two electrodes)

Unipolar lead

- In a unipolar system, the electric current moves from the pulse generator through the lead wire to the negative pole.
- From there, it stimulates the heart and returns to the pulse generator's metal surface (the positive pole) to complete the circuit.

(Text continues on page 250.)

A view of a unipolar lead

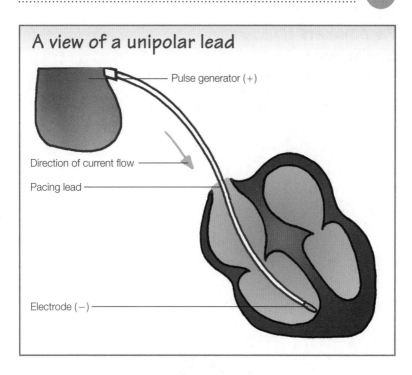

Pulse generator (+)

Direction of current flow

Pacing lead

Electrode (−)

Pacemakers *(continued)*

Bipolar lead

- In a bipolar system, current flows from the pulse generator through the lead wire to the negative pole at the top.
- It stimulates the heart and then flows to the positive pole in the tip to complete the circuit.

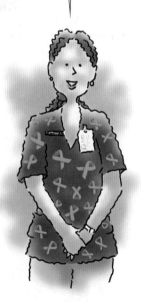

Bipolar systems aren't as easily affected by electrical activity originating outside the heart, such as skeletal muscle contraction and magnetic fields.

(Text continues on page 252.)

A view of a bipolar lead

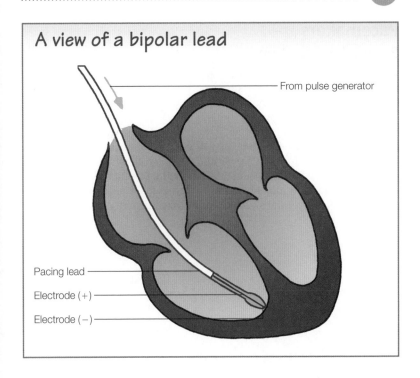

From pulse generator

Pacing lead

Electrode (+)

Electrode (−)

Pacemakers *(continued)*
Pacemaker insertion

- Implanting a pacemaker is a surgical procedure performed with local anesthesia and conscious sedation.
- For lead placement in the atrium, the tip of the catheter must lodge in the right atrium or coronary sinus.
- For placement in the ventricle, it must lodge in the right ventricular apex in one of the interior muscular ridges, or trabeculae.
- When the lead is in correct position, the pulse generator is secured in a subcutaneous pocket of tissue just below the patient's clavicle.
- Changing the generator's battery or microchip circuitry requires a shallow incision over the site and a quick exchange of components.

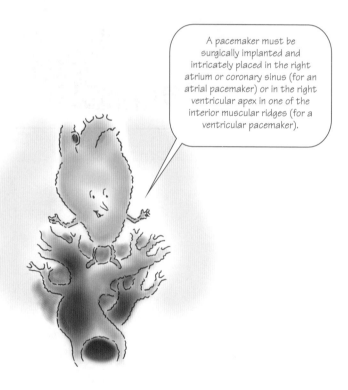

A pacemaker must be surgically implanted and intricately placed in the right atrium or coronary sinus (for an atrial pacemaker) or in the right ventricular apex in one of the interior muscular ridges (for a ventricular pacemaker).

(Text continues on page 254.)

Understanding pacemaker placement

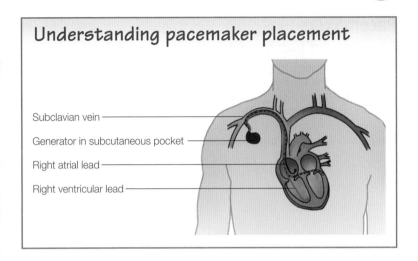

Subclavian vein

Generator in subcutaneous pocket

Right atrial lead

Right ventricular lead

Pacemakers *(continued)*
Biventricular pacemaker

- Uses three leads
    - One to pace the right atrium
    - Another to pace the right ventricle
    - The third to pace the left ventricle
- Paces both ventricles at the same time, causing them to contract simultaneously, which improves cardiac output

> Think about it: if both ventricles contract at the same time, cardiac output improves.

(Text continues on page 256.)

A view of a biventricular lead

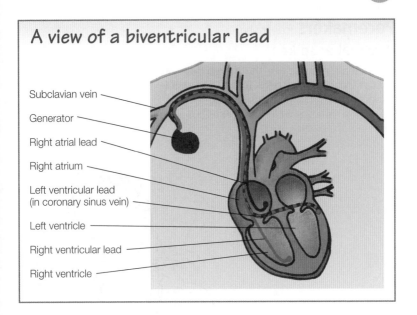

Subclavian vein

Generator

Right atrial lead

Right atrium

Left ventricular lead
(in coronary sinus vein)

Left ventricle

Right ventricular lead

Right ventricle

Pacemakers *(continued)*

Pacemaker spikes

- Pacemaker impulses—the stimuli that travel from the pacemaker to the heart—are visible on the patient's ECG tracing as spikes.
- Large or small, pacemaker spikes appear above or below the isoelectric line.

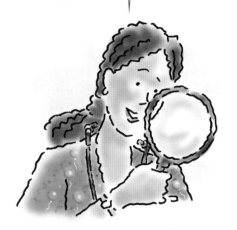

Ah ha! Spikes on a patient's ECG are a tell-tale sign of a pacemaker at work.

(Text continues on page 258.)

Recognizing pacemaker spikes

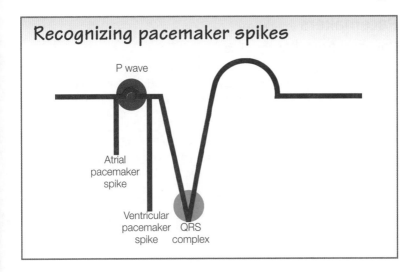

P wave

Atrial
pacemaker
spike

Ventricular
pacemaker   QRS
spike   complex

Pacemakers *(continued)*

Pacemaker spikes *(continued)*

Distinguishing intermittent ventricular pacing from PVCs

● First identify whether the patient has an artificial pacemaker.

● If the monitoring system being used eliminates artifact from ECG tracings, make sure the monitor is set up correctly for a patient with a pacemaker.

● A **paced ventricular complex** will have a pacemaker spike preceding it, as shown in the shaded area on the ECG strip to the right.

● Bipolar pacemaker spikes are small and may be difficult to see, so look in different leads if necessary.

● The paced ventricular complex in a properly functioning pacemaker won't occur early or prematurely; it will only occur when the patient's own ventricular rate falls below the rate set for the pacemaker.

(Text continues on page 260.)

Recognizing intermittent ventricular pacing

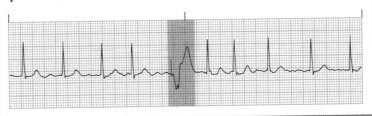

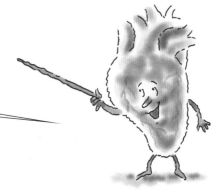

A paced ventricular complex will have a pacemaker spike preceding it, distinguishing it from a PVC.

Pacemakers *(continued)*

Pacemaker spikes *(continued)*

Distinguishing intermittent ventricular pacing from PVCs (continued)

- If the patient is having **PVCs**, they'll occur prematurely.
- Also, they won't have pacemaker spikes preceding them.
- The shaded areas on the ECG to the right show examples of PVCs.

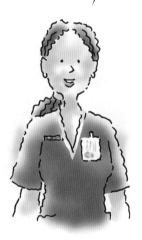

Knowing whether your patient has an artificial pacemaker helps you avoid mistaking a ventricular paced beat for a PVC.

Recognizing PVCs

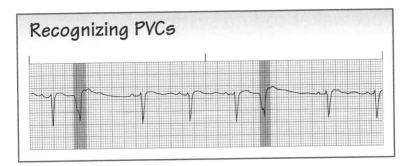

Pacemaker coding systems

- A uniform coding system is used to describe how a pacemaker is programmed.
- The system typically uses three letters to indicate the chamber paced, the chamber sensed, and the response to sensing.
- Pacemaker codes include AAI, VVI, DVI, and DDD.

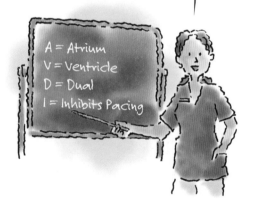

(Text continues on page 264.)

Understanding pacemaker codes

First letter	Second letter	Third letter
Identifies heart chambers that are paced: **V** = Ventricle **A** = Atrium **D** = Dual (ventricle and atrium) **O** = None	Signifies the heart chamber where the pacemaker senses the intrinsic activity: **V** = Ventricle **A** = Atrium **D** = Dual **O** = None	Shows the pacemaker's response to the intrinsic electrical activity it senses in the atrium or ventricle: **T** = Triggers pacing **I** = Inhibits pacing **D** = Dual (can be triggered or inhibited depending on the mode and where intrinsic activity occurs) **O** = None (the pacemaker doesn't change its mode in response to sensed activity)

Pacemaker coding systems *(continued)*

AAI pacemaker

- Is a single-chamber pacemaker
- Consists of an electrode placed in the atrium
- Senses and paces the atria only
- Inhibits pacing and resets itself when it senses intrinsic atrial activity
- QRS complex following pacing results from the heart's own conduction

VVI pacemaker

- Is a single-chamber pacemaker
- Consists of an electrode placed in the ventricle
- Senses and paces the ventricles only
- Used only for patients who don't need atrial kick
- Rhythm is said to reflect 100% pacing when each spike is followed by depolarization, as shown on the bottom strip to the right

(Text continues on page 266.)

ECG effects of AAI and VVI pacemakers

AAI pacemaker

Each atrial spike... ...is followed by a P wave (atrial depolarization).

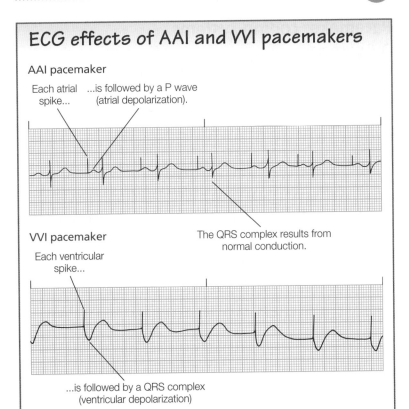

The QRS complex results from normal conduction.

VVI pacemaker

Each ventricular spike...

...is followed by a QRS complex (ventricular depolarization)

Pacemaker coding systems *(continued)*
DVI pacemaker

- Is a dual-chambered pacemaker that paces both the atria and ventricles
- Senses only ventricular intrinsic activity and inhibits ventricular pacing
- *Committed DVI pacemaker:*
    - Generates an impulse even with spontaneous ventricular depolarization
    - Illustrated by the ECG strip to the right
    - Two of the complexes occurred during the AV interval, when the pacemaker was committed to fire
    - As a result, the pacemaker didn't sense the intrinsic QRS complex
- *Noncommitted DVI pacemaker:*
    - Is inhibited if a spontaneous depolarization occurs
    - Spikes won't appear after the QRS complex because the stimulus to pace the ventricles would be inhibited

(Text continues on page 268.)

ECG effects of a DVI pacemaker

The ventricular pacemaker fires despite the intrinsic QRS complex.

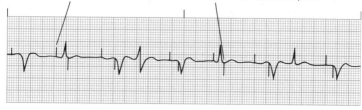

Pacemaker coding systems (continued)

DDD pacemaker

- Set with a rate range rather than a single critical rate
- Senses atrial activity and ensures that the ventricles respond to each atrial stimulation
- Fires when the ventricle doesn't respond on its own
- Paces the atria when the atrial rate falls below the lower set rate
- Illustrated by the ECG strip to the right
  - Complexes 1, 2, 4, and 5 reveal the atrial synchronous mode set at a rate of 70.
  - The patient has an intrinsic P wave so the pacemaker only makes sure the ventricles respond.
  - Complexes 3, 5, 8, 10, and 12 are intrinsic ventricular depolarizations.
  - The pacemaker senses these depolarizations and inhibits firing.
  - In complexes 6, 9, and 11, the pacemaker is pacing both the atria and the ventricles in sequence.
  - In complex 13, only the atria are paced; the ventricles respond on their own.

ECG effects of a DDD pacemaker

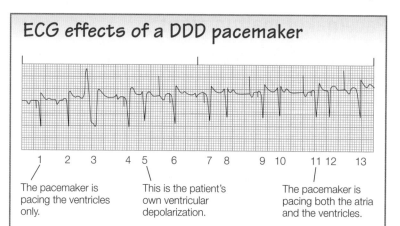

| 1 | 2 | 3 | 4 | 5 | 6 | 7 | 8 | 9 | 10 | 11 | 12 | 13 |

The pacemaker is pacing the ventricles only.

This is the patient's own ventricular depolarization.

The pacemaker is pacing both the atria and the ventricles.

Pacemaker malfunctions

● Malfunction may lead to arrhythmias, hypotension, syncope, and other signs and symptoms of decreased cardiac output.
● Common problems include failure to capture or stimulate the heart chamber, failure to pace or produce activity, and under sensing.

Failure to capture

● Results when the pacemaker fails to stimulate the heart chamber
● Reflected on the ECG by a pacemaker spike without the appropriate atrial or ventricular response (a spike without a complex)
● May occur because of increased pacing thresholds related to:
  – metabolic or electrolyte imbalance
  – antiarrhythmics
  – fibrosis or edema at the pacemaker electrode tip
  – dislodged, broken, or damaged lead
  – perforation of the myocardium by the lead
  – loose connection between the lead and the pulse generator

(Text continues on page 272.)

Recognizing failure to capture

Something's definitely wrong if you see a spike without a response from the heart.

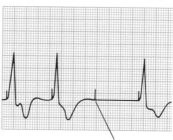

There's a pacemaker spike but no response from the heart.

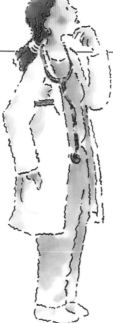

Pacemaker malfunctions (continued)

Failure to pace

- Reflected by an ECG that shows no pacemaker activity when pace-maker activity should be evident
- Also reflected by a lack of response to magnetic application
- May result because of:
  - circuit failure
  - inappropriate programming
  - electromagnetic interference
  - depleted battery

(Text continues on page 274.)

Recognizing failure to pace

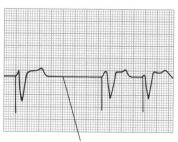

A pacemaker spike should appear here but doesn't.

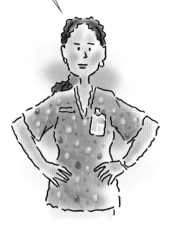

In pacemaker-dependent patients, failure to pace can spell trouble, possibly leading to asystole or a severe decrease in cardiac output.

Pacemaker malfunctions (continued)

Failure to sense intrinsic beats

- Also referred to as undersensing
- Reflected by an ECG that may show pacing spikes anywhere in the cycle, including where intrinsic cardiac activity is present
- May cause the patient to feel palpitations or skipped heart beats
- May trigger ventricular tachycardia or fibrillation if a spike falls on a T wave
- May occur because of:
  - battery failure
  - fracture of the pacing lead wire
  - displacement of the electrode tip
  - "cross-talk" between atrial and ventricular channels
  - electromagnetic interference mistaken for intrinsic signals

Recognizing failure to sense intrinsic beats

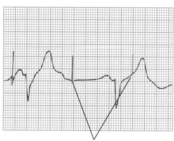

The pacemaker fires anywhere in the cycle.

Replacing the pulse generator battery or lead wires may solve a problem with undersensing.

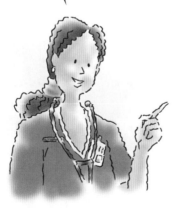

Atlas of Pathophysiology, 3rd ed. Philadelphia: Lippincott Williams & Wilkins, 2009.

Cardiovascular Care Made Incredibly Visual. Philadelphia: Lippincott Williams & Wilkins, 2007.

Cohen, B. *Memmler's Structure and Function of the Human Body*, 9th ed. Philadelphia: Lippincott Williams & Wilkins, 2009.

ECG Interpretation: An Incredibly Easy Workout. Philadelphia: Lippincott Williams & Wilkins, 2008.

ECG Interpretation Made Incredibly Easy, 4th ed. Philadelphia: Lippincott Williams & Wilkins, 2007.

ECG Strip Ease. Philadelphia: Lippincott Williams & Wilkins, 2007.

Interpreting Difficult ECGs: A Rapid Reference. Philadelphia: Lippincott Williams & Wilkins, 2006.

Moses, H.W., and Mullin, J.C. *A Practical Guide to Cardiac Pacing*, 6th ed. Philadelphia: Lippincott Williams & Wilkins, 2007.

Nursing Know-How: Interpreting ECGs. Philadelphia: Lippincott Williams & Wilkins, 2008.

Surawicz, B., and Knilans, T. *Chou's Electrocardiography in Clinical Practice*, 6th ed. Philadelphia: W.B. Saunders, 2008.

A

AAI pacemaker, 264
  ECG effects of, 265i
Abnormalities on rhythm strip, evaluating, 98, 99i
Accelerated junctional rhythm, 146, 147i
Acebutolol, ECG changes with, 236, 237i
Adenosine, ECG changes with, 244, 245i
Amiodarone, ECG changes with, 238, 239i
Angina, 192. *See also* Prinzmetal's angina.
  ECG changes in, 192, 193i
  types of, 192
Anterior-wall MI, 204, 205i
Anteroseptal-wall MI, 206, 207i
Arrhythmias, 104-189
Artifact as monitor problem
  causes of, 50
  identifying, 51i
Asystole, 170, 171i
Atrial arrhythmias, 116-139
Atrial conduction system, 4, 5i
Atrial depolarization, P wave and, 66
Atrial fibrillation, 132, 133i
  distinguishing
    from atrial flutter, 134, 135i
    from junctional rhythm, 138, 139i
    from multifocal atrial tachycardia, 136, 137i
  untreated, complications of, 132
Atrial flutter, 130, 131i
  distinguishing, from atrial fibrillation, 134, 135i
Atrial kick, 116
Atrial rate, determining, on rhythm strip, 86, 87i
Atrial rhythm, evaluating, on rhythm strip, 84, 85i
Atrial standstill, 110
Atrial tachycardia, 120, 121i
  with block, 122, 123i

  distinguishing, from sinus arrhythmia with U waves, 128, 129i
  multifocal, 124, 125i
    distinguishing, from atrial fibrillation, 136, 137i
  paroxysmal, 126, 127i
Atrioventricular block, 174-189
  first-degree, 174, 175i
  third-degree, 182-183i
  type I second-degree, 176-177i
  type II second-degree, 178, 179i
    distinguishing, from nonconducted PATs, 180, 181i
Atrioventricular node, 6
  conduction system and, 3i, 4, 6, 7i
AV block. *See* Atrioventricular block.
AV node. *See* Atrioventricular node.

B

Bachmann's bundle, 4, 5i
Beta-adrenergic blockers, ECG changes with, 236, 237i
Bigeminy, 156, 157i
Bipolar leads, 10, 11i
  in pacemaker, 250, 251i
Bundle branch block, 184-189
  distinguishing, from Wolff-Parkinson-White syndrome, 188, 189i
  left, 184, 186, 187i
  right, 184, 185i
Bundle branches, ventricular conduction and, 6, 7i
Bundle of His, ventricular conduction and, 6, 7i

C

Calcium channel blockers, ECG changes with, 240, 241i
Cardiac cells, polarized, 2
Cardiac drugs, ECG changes with, 230-245
Class IA antiarrhythmics, ECG changes with, 230, 231i

Note: t refers to a table; i refers to an illustration.

Class IB antiarrhythmics, ECG changes with, 232, 233i
Class IC antiarrhythmics, ECG changes with, 234, 235i
Class II antiarrhythmics, ECG changes with, 236, 237i
Class III antiarrhythmics, ECG changes with, 238, 239i
Class IV antiarrhythmics, ECG changes with, 240, 241i
Classifying rhythm strip characteristics, 98, 99i
Complete heart block, 182, 183i
Conduction system, 2-7

D
DDD pacemaker, 268
    ECG effects of, 269i
Depolarization, 2
Digoxin, ECG changes with, 242, 243i
Digoxin toxicity
    ST segment in, 76, 77i
    U wave and, 82
Diltiazem, ECG changes with, 240, 241i
DVI pacemaker, 266
    ECG effects of, 267i

E
ECG changes
    with adenosine, 244, 245i
    in angina, 192, 193i
    with calcium channel blockers, 240, 241i
    with class IA antiarrhythmics, 230, 231i
    with class IB antiarrhythmics, 232, 233i
    with class IC antiarrhythmics, 234, 235i
    with class II antiarrhythmics, 236, 237i
    with class III antiarrhythmics, 238, 239i
    with class IV antiarrhythmics, 240, 241i
    with digoxin, 242, 243i
    in hypercalcemia, 226, 227i
    in hyperkalemia, 222, 223i
    in hypocalcemia, 228, 229i
    in hypokalemia, 224, 225i
    in infarction stage of MI, 198, 199i
    in injury stage of MI, 196, 197i
    in ischemia stage of MI, 196, 197i
    in left ventricular hypertrophy, 218, 219i
    in pericarditis, 214, 215i
    in Prinzmetal's angina, 194, 195i
ECG complex, components of, 64-84, 65i. See also specific component.
ECG evaluation, 8-step method of, 84-99
ECG printout, 44, 45i
    horizontal axis blocks on, 46, 47i
    vertical axis blocks on, 48, 49i
Electrolyte imbalances, ECG changes in, 222-229
Esmolol, ECG changes with, 236, 237i

F
Failure to capture as pacemaker malfunction, 270, 271i
Failure to pace as pacemaker malfunction, 272, 273i
Failure to sense intrinsic beats as pacemaker malfunction, 274, 275i
False high-rate alarm as monitor problem causes of, 52
    identifying, 53i
Fascicular block, 184
Fibrillatory waves, 134, 135i
First-degree AV block, 174, 175i
Flecainide, ECG changes with, 234, 235i
Flutter waves, 134, 135i
Frontal plane of heart, 14, 15i
Fuzzy baseline as monitor problem causes of, 58
    identifying, 59i
F waves, 134, 135i

H
Hemiblock, 184
His-Purkinje system repolarization, U wave and, 82
Horizontal axis blocks on ECG printout, 46, 47i
Horizontal plane of heart, 14, 15i
Hypercalcemia
    ECG changes in, 226, 227i
    U wave and, 82
Hyperkalemia, ECG changes in, 222, 223i

Note: t refers to a table; i refers to an illustration.

Hypocalcemia, ECG changes in, 228, 229i
Hypokalemia
ECG changes in, 224, 225i
U wave and, 82

I

Ibutilide, ECG changes with, 238, 239i
Idioventricular arrhythmia, 158, 159i
accelerated, 160, 161i
Infarction stage of MI, ECG changes in, 198, 199i
Inferior-wall MI, 208, 209i
Injury stage of MI, ECG changes in, 196, 197i
Interatrial tract, conduction through, 4, 5i
Intermittent ventricular pacing, distinguishing, from PVCs, 258, 259i, 260, 261i
Internodal tracts, conduction system and, 4, 5i
Ischemia stage of MI, ECG changes in, 196, 197i
Isoelectric deflection, 8

JK

J point, 65i, 74
Junctional arrhythmias, 140-151
variations in P wave position in, 140, 141i
Junctional escape rhythm, 144, 145i
Junctional rhythm, distinguishing, from atrial fibrillation, 138, 139i
Junctional tachycardia, 148, 149i

L

Lateral-wall MI, 210, 211i
Lead I limb lead, 16, 17i
Lead II limb lead, 18, 19i
Lead III limb lead, 20, 21i
Lead aV_F limb lead, 26, 27i
Lead aV_L limb lead, 24, 25i
Lead aV_R limb lead, 22, 23i
Lead V_1 precordial lead, 28, 29i
Lead V_2 precordial lead, 30, 31i
Lead V_3 precordial lead, 32, 33i
Lead V_4 precordial lead, 34, 35i
Lead V_5 precordial lead, 36, 37i

Lead V_6 precordial lead, 38, 39i
Leads
axis of, 8
bipolar, 10, 11i
in pacemaker, 250, 251i
limb, 16, 17i, 18, 19i, 20, 21i, 22, 23i, 24, 25i, 26, 27i
modified chest, 40, 41i, 42, 43i
precordial, 28, 29i, 30, 31i, 32, 33i, 34, 35i, 36, 37i, 38, 39i
unipolar, 12, 13i
in pacemaker, 248, 249i
Left bundle branch block, 186, 187i
Left ventricular hypertrophy, ECG changes in, 218, 219i
Lidocaine, ECG changes with, 232, 233i
Limb leads, 16-27

M

MAT. See Multifocal atrial tachycardia.
MCL_1, 40, 41i
MCL_6, 42, 43i
Mexiletine, ECG changes with, 232, 233i
MI. See Myocardial infarction.
Mobitz I block, 176, 177i
Mobitz II block. See Type II second-degree AV block.
Modified chest leads, 40-43
Monitor problems, identifying, 50-61
Moricizine, ECG changes with, 234, 235i
Multifocal atrial tachycardia, 124, 125i
distinguishing, from atrial fibrillation, 136, 137i
Multiform premature ventricular contractions, 154, 155i
Myocardial infarction, 196-213
anterior-wall, 204, 205i
anteroseptal-wall, 206, 207i
distinguishing, from acute pericarditis, 216, 217i
ECG changes
in infarction stage, 198, 199i
in injury stage, 196, 197i
in ischemia stage, 196, 197i
inferior-wall, 208, 209i
ischemia in, 196, 197i
lateral-wall, 210, 211i
locating damage in, 202, 203t

Note: t refers to a table; i refers to an illustration.

reciprocal changes in, 200, 201i
right-ventricular-wall, 212, 213i
Myocardial injury, ST segment in, 76, 77i
Myocardial ischemia, ST segment in, 76, 77i

NO

Normal sinus rhythm, 100, 101i

P

Paced ventricular complex, 258, 259i, 260, 261i
Pacemaker coding systems, 262, 263t, 264-269
Pacemakers, 248-275
  AAI, 264, 265i
  bipolar system for, 250, 251i
  biventricular, 254, 255i
  DDD, 268, 269i
  DVI, 266, 267i
  inserting, 252
  lead placement for, 252, 253i
  malfunctions of, 270-275
  unipolar system for, 248, 249i
  VVI, 264, 265i
Pacemaker spikes, 256-261
Paired PVCs, 154, 155i
Paroxysmal atrial tachycardia, 126, 127i
PATs. See Premature atrial contractions.
Pericarditis
  acute, distinguishing, from myocardial infarction, 216, 217i
  ECG changes in, 214, 215i
Phenytoin, ECG changes with, 232, 233i
Planes of heart, 14, 15i
Potassium channel blockers, ECG changes with, 238, 239i
Precordial leads, 28-39
Premature atrial contractions, 116, 117i
  nonconducted, distinguishing
    from SA block, 118, 119i
    from type II second-degree AV block, 180, 181i
Premature junctional contractions, 142, 143i
Premature ventricular contractions, 152, 153i
  bigeminy and, 156, 157i

distinguishing, from intermittent ventricular pacing, 258, 259i, 260, 261i
  multiform, 154, 155i
  paired, 154, 155i
  R-on-T phenomenon and, 156, 157i
  trigeminy and, 156, 157i
PR interval, 65i, 68, 69i
  calculating, on rhythm strip, 90, 91i
Prinzmetal's angina, 194. See also Angina.
  ECG changes in, 194, 195i
Procainamide, ECG changes with, 230, 231i
Propafenone, ECG changes with, 234, 235i
Propranolol, ECG changes with, 236, 237i
Pulseless electrical activity, 172, 173i
Purkinje fibers, 6, 7i
P wave, 65i, 66, 67i
  evaluating, on rhythm strip, 88, 89i
  variations in position of, in junctional arrhythmias, 140, 141i

Q

QRS complex, 65i, 70, 71i
  calculating duration of, on rhythm strip, 92, 93i
  waveform variations in, 72, 73i
QT interval, 65i, 80, 81i
  determining, on rhythm strip, 96, 97i
Quinidine, ECG changes with, 230, 231i
Q wave, 65i, 70, 71i

R

Rate
  classifying, on rhythm strip, 98
  determining, in ECG evaluation, 86, 87i
Repolarization, 2
Rhythm
  classifying, on rhythm strip, 98
  determining, in ECG evaluation, 84, 85i
  origin of, classifying, on rhythm strip, 98
Rhythm of last resort, 158, 159i
Rhythm strip interpretation, 64-101

Note: t refers to a table; i refers to an illustration.

Right bundle branch block, 184, 185i
Right-ventricular-wall MI, 212, 213i
R-on-T phenomenon, 156, 157i
R wave, 65i, 70, 71i

S

SA block, 112, 113i
  distinguishing, from nonconducted
    PATs, 118, 119i
SA node. *See* Sinoatrial node.
Sick sinus syndrome, 114, 115i
Sinoatrial exit block, 112, 113i
Sinoatrial node, 2, 4, 5i, 104. *See also*
    Sinus node arrhythmias.
Sinus arrest, 110, 111i
Sinus arrhythmia, 104, 105i
  with U waves, distinguishing, from
    atrial tachycardia with block,
    128, 129i
Sinus bradycardia, 106, 107i
Sinus node arrhythmias, 104-115
  causes of, 104
Sinus pause, 110, 115i
Sinus tachycardia, 108, 109i
Sotalol, ECG changes with, 238, 239i
ST segment, 65i, 74, 75i
  changes in, 76, 77i
S wave, 65i, 70, 71i

T

Tachycardia
  atrial, 120, 121i
  junctional, 148, 149i
  sinus, 108, 109i
  ventricular, 162, 163i
Third-degree AV block, 182, 183i
Torsades de pointes, 164, 165i
  distinguishing, from ventricular flutter,
    166, 167i
Trigeminy, 156
T wave, 65i, 78, 79i
  evaluating, on rhythm strip, 94, 95i
Type I second-degree AV block, 176, 177i
Type II second-degree AV block, 178, 179i
  distinguishing, from nonconducted
    PATs, 180, 181i

U

Undersensing as pacemaker malfunc-
    tion, 274, 275i
Unipolar leads, 12, 13i
  in pacemaker, 248, 249i
U wave, 65i, 82, 83i

V

Ventricular arrhythmias, 152-168
Ventricular conduction, QRS complex
    and, 70
Ventricular conduction system, 6, 7i
Ventricular couplet, 154, 155i
Ventricular fibrillation, 168, 169i
Ventricular flutter, distinguishing, from
    torsades de pointes, 166, 167i
Ventricular rate, determining, on rhythm
    strip, 86, 87i
Ventricular rhythm, evaluating, on rhythm
    strip, 84, 85i
Ventricular tachycardia, 162, 163i
Verapamil, ECG changes with, 240, 241i
Vertical axis blocks on ECG printout,
    48, 49i
VVI pacemaker, 264
  ECG effect of, 265i

WXYZ

Wandering baseline as monitor problem
  causes of, 56
  identifying, 57i
Waveform
  absent, as monitor problem
    causes of, 60
    identifying, 61i
  deflection of, 8, 9i
  variations of, in QRS complex, 72, 73i
Waveform interference. *See* Artifact.
Weak signals as monitor problem
  causes of, 54
  identifying, 55i
Wenckebach block, 176, 177i
Wolff-Parkinson-White syndrome, 150,
    151i
  distinguishing, from bundle branch
    block, 188, 189i

RRS0904

Note: t refers to a table; i refers to an illustration.